HOME WORKOUTS

HOW TO STAY FIT
JUST BY USING YOUR OWN BODY WEIGHT

ATHANASIOS NANOS

2020

To my daughter, Dimitra

Published in 2020
Book Series: Workouts for Ordinary People.

Copyright ©: Athanasios Nanos

Text Editing: Katerina Ampatzi

Design and composition: Athanasios Nanos

contact: mikelonere@gmail.com

ISBN: 979-865-29-4896-2

Contents

Few things about me...5

Introduction...6

Quick guide for Home Workouts...7

Health and Safety Issues...8

Benefits of Workout...9

Heart rate and Workouts...10

Useful Tips for creating the best workout space...11

Stretching Exercises...12

Importance of Stretching Exercises...13

Stretching Techniques...14

Stretching Exercises...15

Workouts, repeats and sets...19

PART ONE / LEVELS 1-6 (Workouts for core and upper body muscles)...20

How it works...21

Tips for LEVEL 1-6 Workouts...22

LEVEL 1...24

LEVEL 2...25

LEVEL 3...26

LEVEL 4...27

LEVEL 5...28

LEVEL 6...29

PART TWO / LEVELS 7-11 (Workouts for lower body muscles)...30

Tips for LEVEL 7-11 Workouts...31

LEVEL 7...32

LEVEL 8...33

LEVEL 9...34

LEVEL 10...35

LEVEL 11...36

PART THREE / LEVELS 12-15 (HIIT Workouts)...37

Tips for HIIT Workouts...38

HIIT Workouts / Basic Rules...39

Squat Jump...40

Push ups...41

Lunges workouts...42

Triceps in Bench...43

Stair Climbing or Step Jumps...44

Skipping Run (fast)...45

Burpees...46

HIIT WORKOUTS...47

HIIT Workouts 1-2-3 Comparison...48

HIIT Workouts 1...49

HIIT Workouts 2...50

HIIT Workouts 3...51

LEVEL 12...52

LEVEL 13...53

LEVEL 14...54

LEVEL 15...55

NOTES...56

Notes Example for LEVELS 1-6,7-11,12-15...57

Notes for LEVELS 1-6...58

Notes for LEVELS 7-11...59

Notes for LEVELS 12-15...60

Few things about me

My name is Athanasios Nanos. I have graduated from the Department of Physical Education and Sports Science of the Aristotle University Of Thessaloniki, Greece, and subsequently I have received a Master of Education by the Department of Primary Education of the University of West Macedonia, Greece. I have been active in sports and physical activities for many years. I have been involved in sport business in a variety of ways: as an athlete, coach, trainer and organizer, club member. Over the last years I have been working as a Teacher of Physical Education in Secondary Education (student ages 12-18) and occupying myself as coach/trainer to Volleyball, Tennis and Water-ski clubs for many years. The result of this accumulated knowledge is offered to you through the present book.

Introduction

Preparing the body and mind for a basic level of fitness can be a really big challenge for anybody. When you perform workouts, your muscular system should be able to sustain exercises without any problem. A basic level of fitness can reduce the chances of injury, protect your health and improve your mental and physical well-being.

You constantly hear people claim that there is no time for workouts. Others find impossible to follow a particular fitness routine. When they are asked to provide possible reasons that discourage them from participating in workouts, they answer:

- really tight daily schedule,
- limited free time,
- family responsibilities,
- long- lasting studying,
- frequent trips,
- long-term absence from workouts/ fear of failure if they start exercising again,
- financial reasons (many are not willing to prepay multi-month gym membership fees that will hardly join).

Time schedules might be tight, but this is not the problem. Statistics show that an average person spends more than five hours on a smartphone during a daily period. However, workouts require less than 30 minutes per day. The duration of the particular workout LEVELS do not last more than 30 minutes (including stretching exercises). The beginning of these workouts could be the beginning of a beautiful journey. It is up to you to change your daily habits and start working out again.

The suggested workouts included in this book are mainly for home use. The exercises are carefully chosen for being performed at home conditions, taking into account the limited space and other peculiarities of the house.

Why workout at home? Because:

- you do not waste a lot of time by moving to the gym,
- you can do workouts at any available time,
- you can daily exercise yourself and can be the coach/trainer of yourself,
- the workouts and program of the present book can help you design a program that fits to your individual needs,
- you can workout at your own pace, based on your needs,
- it is the best way to stay fit even if difficult situations occur (e.g. COVID-19).

Quick guide for Home Workouts

- You will have reached a satisfying level of fitness when you manage to complete LEVEL 15.
- The shortest period of successfully executing LEVELS 1-15 is fifteen (15) weeks. In case you find it really hard to follow workouts of a particular LEVEL, you are kindly requested to repeat the same LEVEL for one week or more. Keep in mind that your goal is to perform exercises properly and not as fast as you can. In some cases this means that you might need to spend more time than a fifteen week period.
- You will repeat workouts of LEVEL 6 three times per week for the following LEVELS 7-15.
- You should write down the number of workouts you do so as to monitor your progress. The tables found on the following pages after LEVEL 15 could be really helpful.
- You can perform cardio workouts if you wish (like running, cycling and intense walking) parallel to the Part 1, Part 2 and Part 3 workouts, as long as the extra cardio workouts do not affect the quality of the LEVELS' workouts.
- You should not worry if you are not able to perform the suggested exercises within the time limit given. Provided that you are capable of executing a particular LEVEL effortlessly, you can carry on with the remaining exercises any time you want during the day or alternatively, you can cover the number of repetitions whenever you wish within a week. Consequently, you can deviate from the suggested plan of executing a particular LEVEL, on condition that you are fit enough to perform the exercises included in this LEVEL.

Home Workouts consists of three parts.

Ø **Part 1 (LEVEL 1 to 6).** Arms and core workouts.

Ø **Part 2 (LEVEL 7-11).** Legs and core workouts.

Ø **Part 3 (LEVEL 12-15).** High Intensive Internal Training (HIIT) workouts.

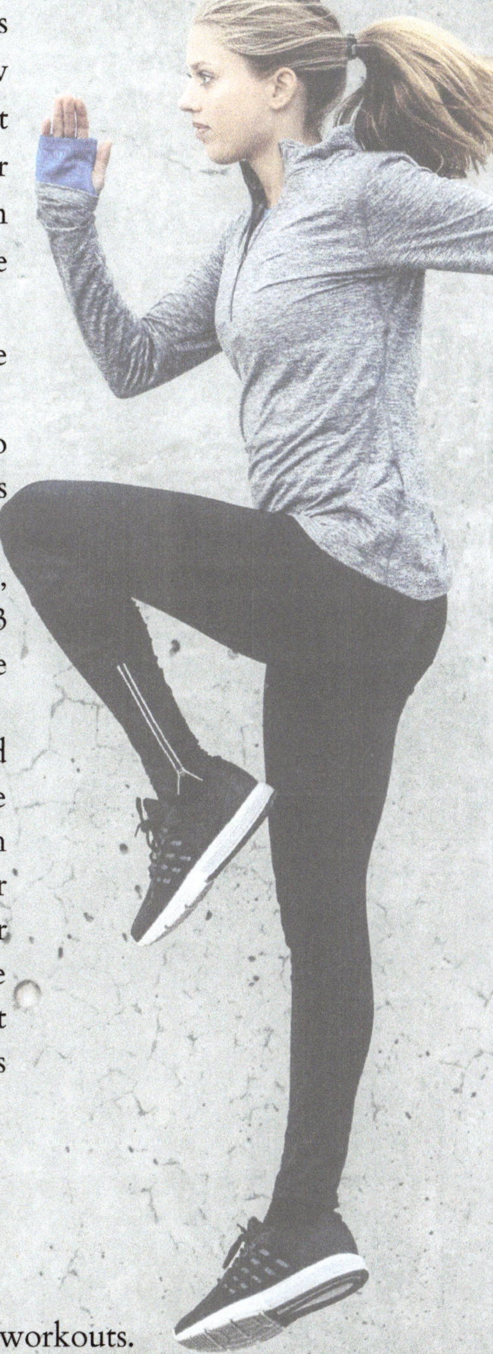

Health and Safety Issues

1.   Before you start to exercise, it is important for you to consult your doctor. A general check with your doctor is suggested by health experts (Mayo Clinic, American College of Sports Medicine) before starting an exercise program, especially if any of the following applies:

- heart disease,
- type I(1) or type II(2) diabetes,
- kidney disease,
- arthritis,
- treated for cancer or recently completed cancer treatment,
- high blood pressure,
- you are over >40 years old,
- you are pregnant,
- you have other health problems.

2.   If a long period has passed since your last workout it is better to check with your doctor, particularly if any of the following symptoms occur:

- pain or discomfort in chest, jaw, arms or neck during exercise or at rest,
- dizziness, lightheadeness, fainting while exercising, shortness of breath on mild exertion at rest, when lying down or going to bed,
- ankle swelling,
- rapid or pronounced heartbeat,
- heart murmur (especially if your doctor has previously heard it),
- any pains (i.e. lower leg pain) that occur when walking, which go away in a state of rest.

Workouts in this book are carefully planned for a moderate physical activity. If in any case you do not feel well with the workouts, it is strongly recommended to stop exercising and visit a doctor.

BENEFITS OF WORKOUT

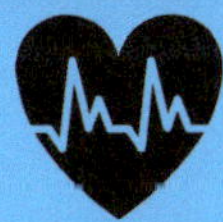 **Exercise will improve your overall health and fitness!**

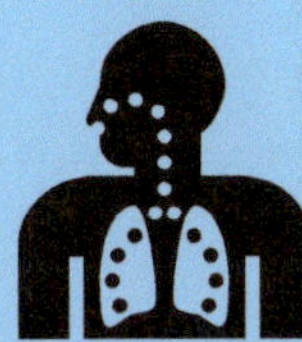 **Exercise will improve your daily life quality!**

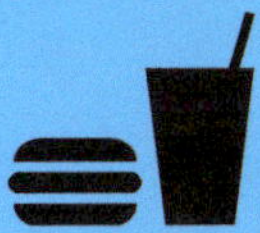 **Exercise will increase metabolism and reduce weight!**

 **Exercise will make you feel happier! With exercise you can dismiss and control the levels of stress and anxiety!**

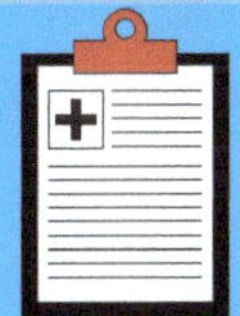 **Exercise will reduce the risk of chronic deseases! Lack of exercise is a primary cause of chronic deseases!**

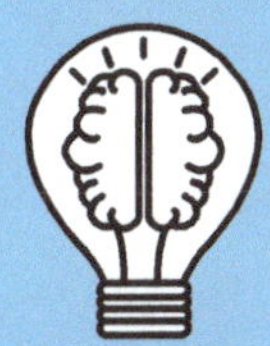 **Exercise will imrove your brain health and memory!**

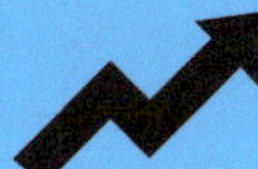 **Exercise will help you live longer!**

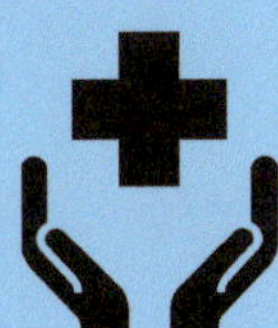 **Overall, you can take the control of the quality of your life by exercising!**

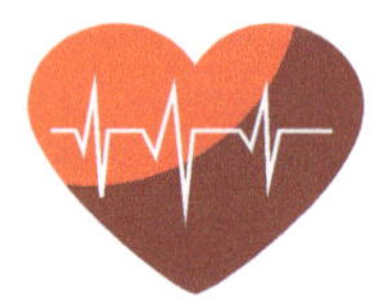

Heart rate and Workouts

Maximum Heart Rate (HRmax) can be calculated by subtracting your age from 220 (heart rate) – age (minus your age). This means that Maximum Heart Rate (HRmax) varies, depending on the age of the participant. For example, HRmax of a twenty (20) year old participant in a HRmax workout is: 220-20 =200. For a forty (40) year old (40) is: 220-40=180 respectively. The intensity of a moderate workout activity covers 50-70% of the HRmax Zone, while intensity of the vigorous workout activity covers 70-85% of the HRmax Zone. In the following table you can see the Heart Rate Zone for the age group of 20 to 70 years.

Age	Target Heart Rate Zone (50-85%) (beats per minute)	Maximum Heart Rate Zone (100%) (beats per minute)
20	100-170	200
30	95-162	190
35	93-157	185
40	90-153	180
45	88-149	175
50	85-145	170
55	83-140	165
60	80-136	160
65	78-132	155
70	75-128	150

Table of Heart Rate Zones

The Heart Rate can be measured by an activity tracker. If there is no activity tracker, you measure your heart rate manually. Take your pulse on the inside of your wrist, on the thumb side. With the tips of the first two fingers press the artery. There are many ways now to measure your heart rate. You can count your pulse for 15 seconds and multiply by four (15"x4= 1'). This will give you beats per minute. But the most precise way is to count pulse for 30 seconds and multiply by two (30"x2 =1').

Heart rate can be the most precise tool for understanding the proper level of pressure when you exercise. If you are a beginner, setting a target zone of 50% of Maximum Heart Rate is satisfactory for you. As time passes and you practice further you will be able to work comfortably at levels close to 85% of the target Heart Rate Zone.

Useful tips for creating the best Workout space

1. Define a space.

You should think about the exercises that you will follow during the workout program. Decide on how much space you will need. You should have enough room to lay an exercise mat down. If the workouts require more intense movements, you may need some more space. Watch out if the room has got low ceilings.

2. Health and safety.

Before starting the workouts, your space should meet the basic safety requirements, meaning: no objects around you that can hurt you during your workout, no objects that could fell on you, be sure to have an exercise mat and avoid slippery floor during intense workout.

3. Create the right atmosphere.

Find the room that you will feel more comfortable for exercising. The exercise should not feel like punishment. You must have a good mood for achieving the workout goals. Clear your space (in order not to be distracted during workouts) and decorate it in a way that will make you feel comfortable and inspired (put pictures, quotes, paintings artwork). A good option is to have a mirror close to you: first you can see if you perform the workouts in the properly way and also it can make a small space to look larger.

4. Keep your space organized.

If you manage to create the workout space as wanted, now the challenge is to keep it clean and organized. That will make your space look attractive and inviting for a new set of workouts. Any equipment is good to keep it close to the workout space (i.e. workout mat), for accessing directly when you need it.

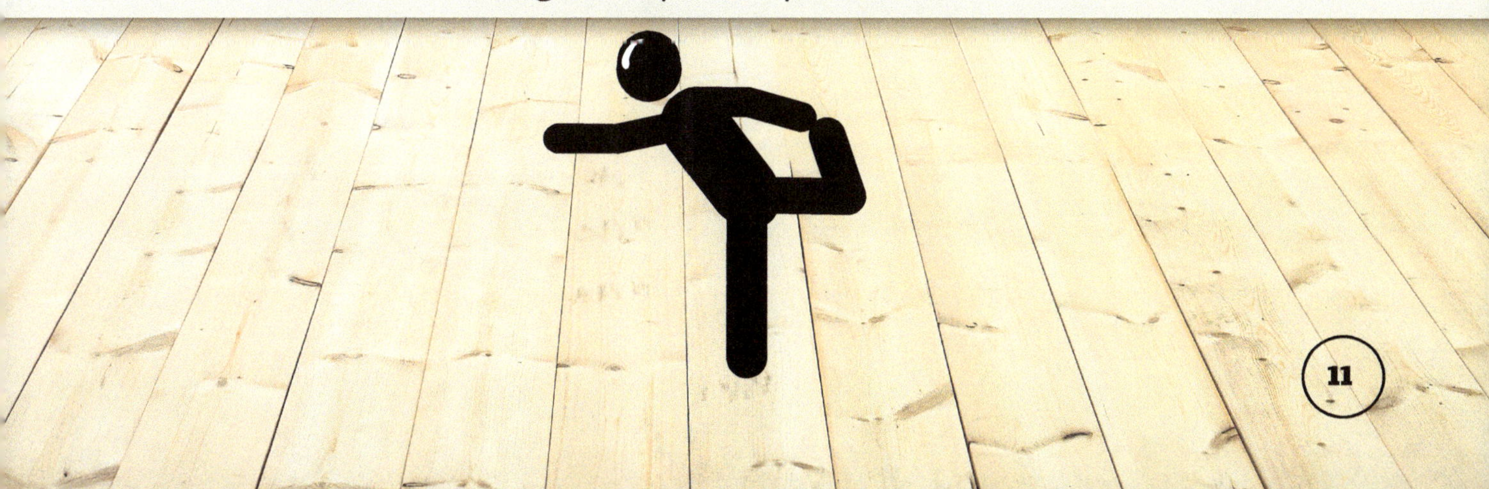

Stretching Exercises

Importance of stretching exercises

Many people might be thinking that stretching is only performed by athletes. Some spend a lot of time in workouts for increasing the level of their strength, without using 10-15 minutes for stretching exercises. The truth is that stretching exercises are really important for many reasons. First of all, they are essential for the well-being of the body. Furthermore, they contribute to each individual's health and the flexibility of his/her muscles.

If you have had a long period without stretching exercises, you will notice that the muscles tend to shorten and can become really tight. When it comes to workouts, the short and tight muscles could have a strong effect on exercise. The muscles are unable to give a full-extent, which in turn will affect the quality of the exercise. Having short and tight muscles can increase the risk of injuries, including muscle damage and joint pains.

A muscular system with high flexibility and elasticity has many advantages:
- stronger muscle contraction during workouts,
- smaller chances of body injuries,
- body can experience a full range of movements during workouts.

You should not expect that your flexibility will be improved with just a day of stretching workouts. You should perform stretching exercises on a daily basis and you will experience a rapid improvement of your elasticity. Even if you reach at the desired level of flexibility, stretching exercises must continue to be a part of your daily workout program. This will ensure that you will retain your muscle flexibility and elasticity at the desired level while stretching exercises will help you avoid injuries before, during and after workouts.

Stretching Techniques

The static stretching exercises are the most suitable type of stretching exercises when you workout at home. Stretching exercises can be really helpful as long as you use the right technique.

Start slowly at the beginning without rushing. You should stretch up to the level that you will start feeling a stretched muscle with a slight discomfort in your muscle. That is your stretching point and hold to it for at least 15 seconds.

The stretching exercises must follow a certain routine order. In this book we start stretching from the top, move to hands and shoulders, body core and finish by stretching our leg muscles. You should avoid exercises without a certain order like starting from the body core, move to the legs and then return again to the body core. Routine order will help you remember to stretch all your body muscles.

You can stretch both before and after workouts. This will help you to get your body system ready, increase your elasticity and protect you from injuries. If you do not have the time to stretch before and after workouts, prefer to stretch after workouts.

Usual mistakes that people make:
- They push more than the desired stretching point and they might cause a muscle injury.
- When they feel discomfort, they loosen up the stretching muscle to a point that no stretching works.
- They keep moving repeatedly from stretching point to loosen up point and back during workout. No stretching improvement will occur. I could describe it as if someone is starting the engine and the moment the engine is about to work he shuts it down. And that is being repeated for several times.

Stretching Exercises

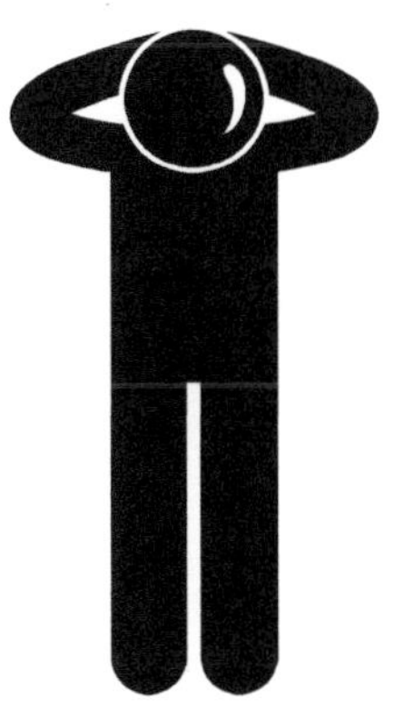

Pushing head down for
for fifteen (15") seconds.

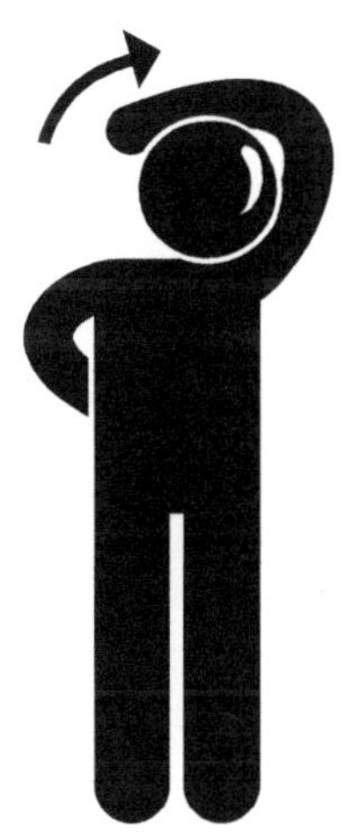

Pushing head to the left
for fifteen (15") seconds.

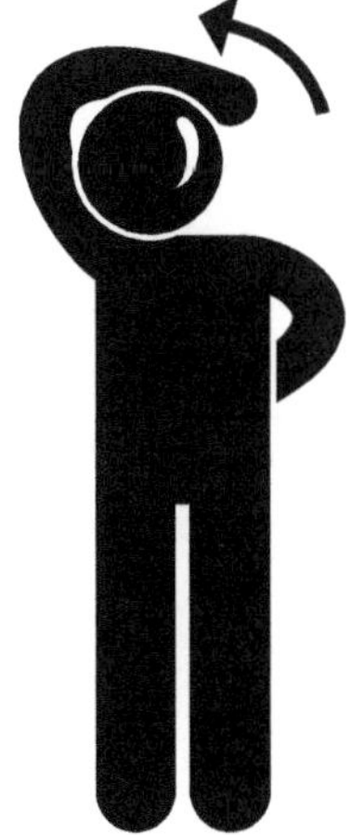

Pushing head to the right
for for fifteen (15") seconds.

Stretching Exercises

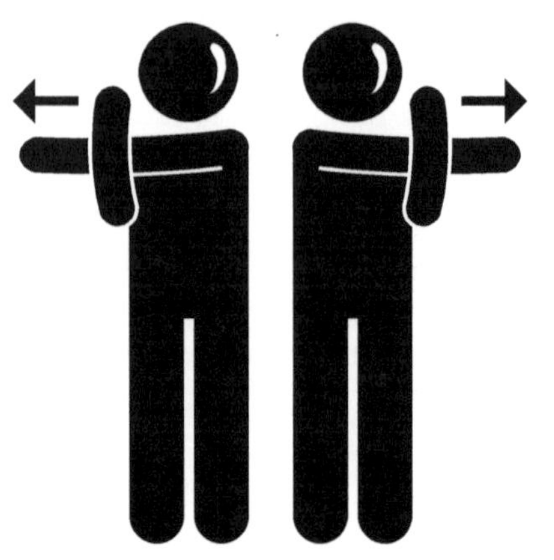

Pushing hands in turn. Pressure is applied to the elbow area. Stretching duration: fifteen (15") seconds for each hand.

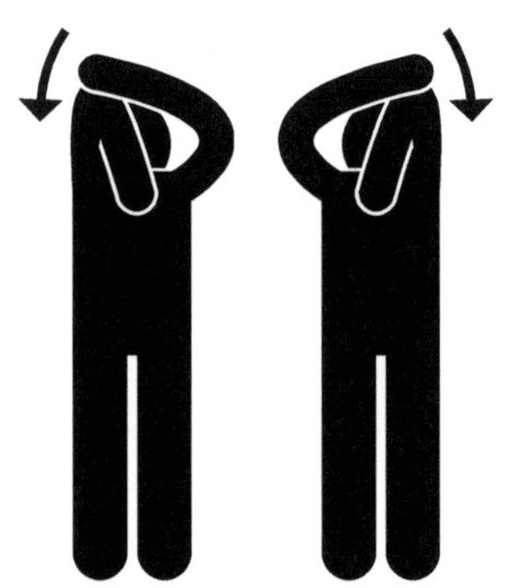

Pushing hands in turn. Pressure is applied to the elbow area. Direction of stretching: as shown left with arrows. Stretching duration: fifteen (15") seconds for each hand.

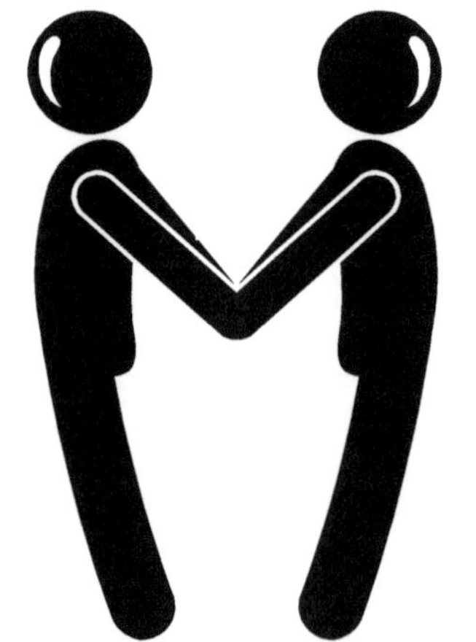

Hand grip at a fixed point or holding the hands of another person. Overxtension of body core. Stretching duration: fifteen (15") seconds.

Stretching Exercises

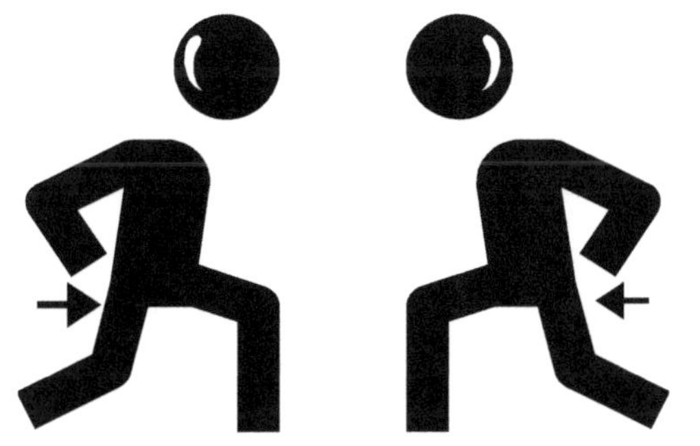

Stretching iliopsoas. Place one leg in front, the other moves back (both soles touch wholesurface during the workout). Push the area of hip bones to the front, without moving your feet. Fifteen (15") seconds of stretching on each foot.

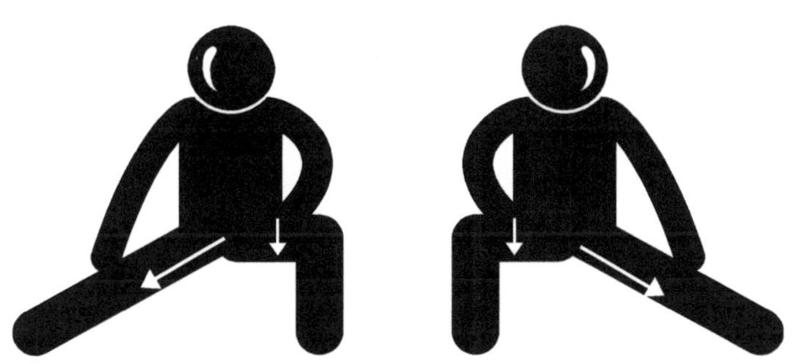

Adductor longus stretching. Fifteen (15") seconds of stretching on each foot.

Biceps femoris stretching. Leg is placed on a bench. The core bends towards the knee. Fifteen (15") seconds of stretching on each foot.

Stretching Exercises

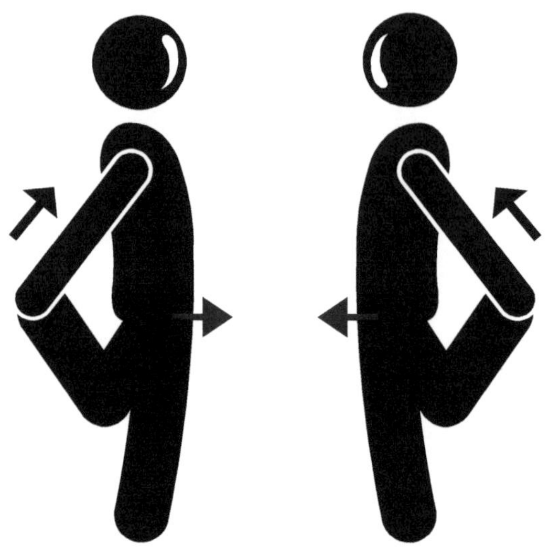

Quadriceps stretching in turn. The hand is pulling back while area of hip bones is pushing infront, as shown in picture. Stretching duration: fifteen (15") seconds.

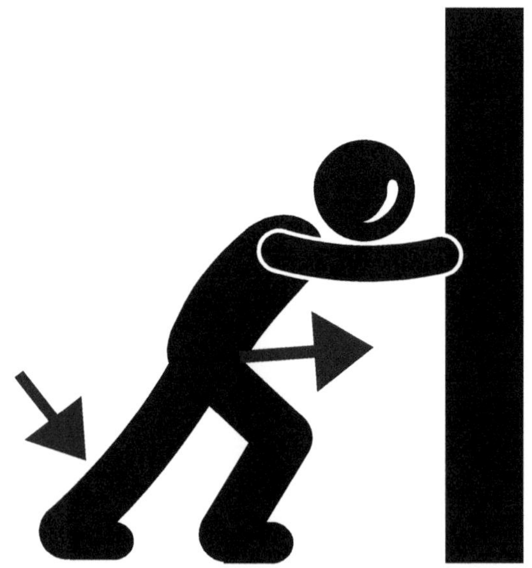

Calf stretching in turn. Stabilize your back foot in surface, while body core pushes towards the wall. Stretching duration: fifteen (15") seconds.

Workouts, repeats and sets

A set is a group of consecutive workouts

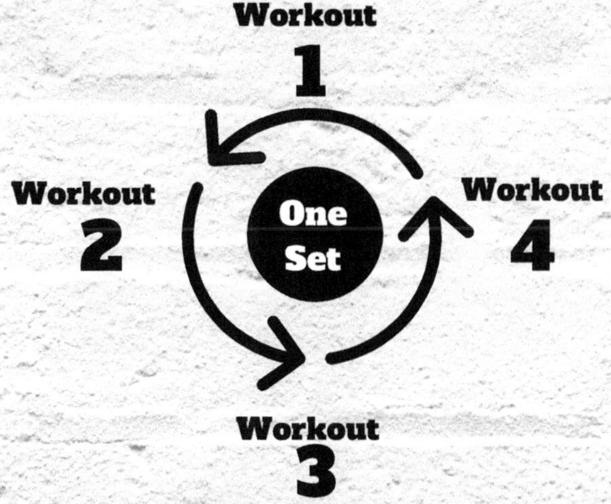

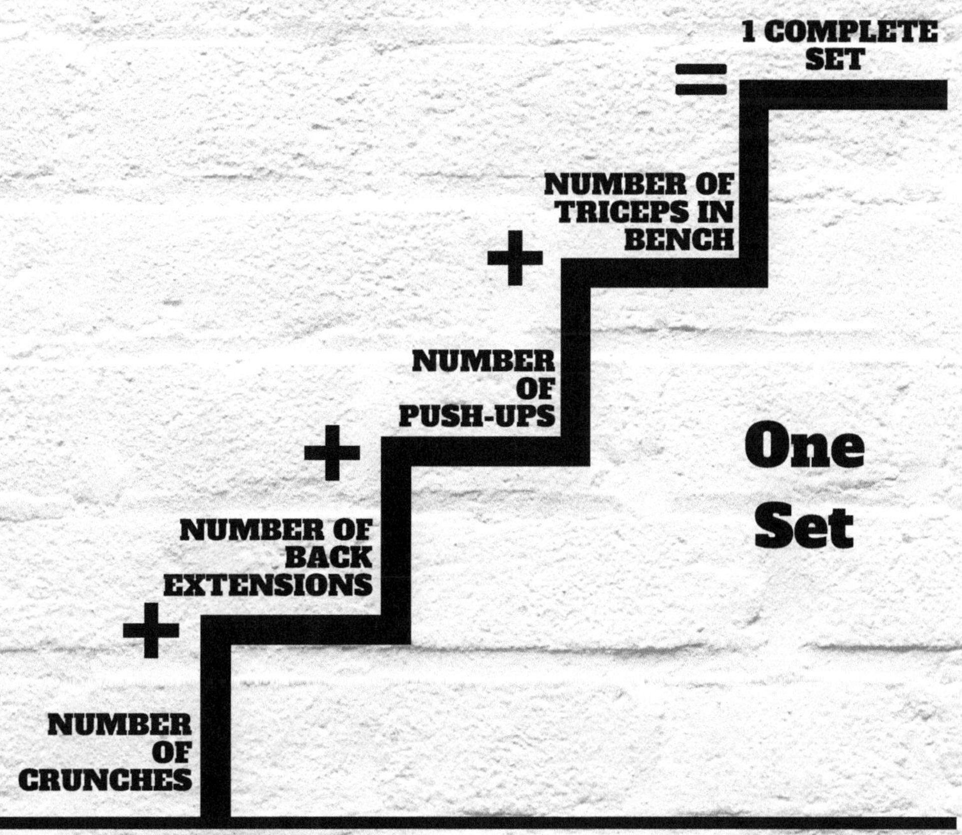

1 COMPLETE SET $\times$ NUMBER OF TIMES = A COMPLETE LEVEL OF WORKOUTS

Part 1
LEVELS 1-6

Workouts for core and upper body muscles

How it works

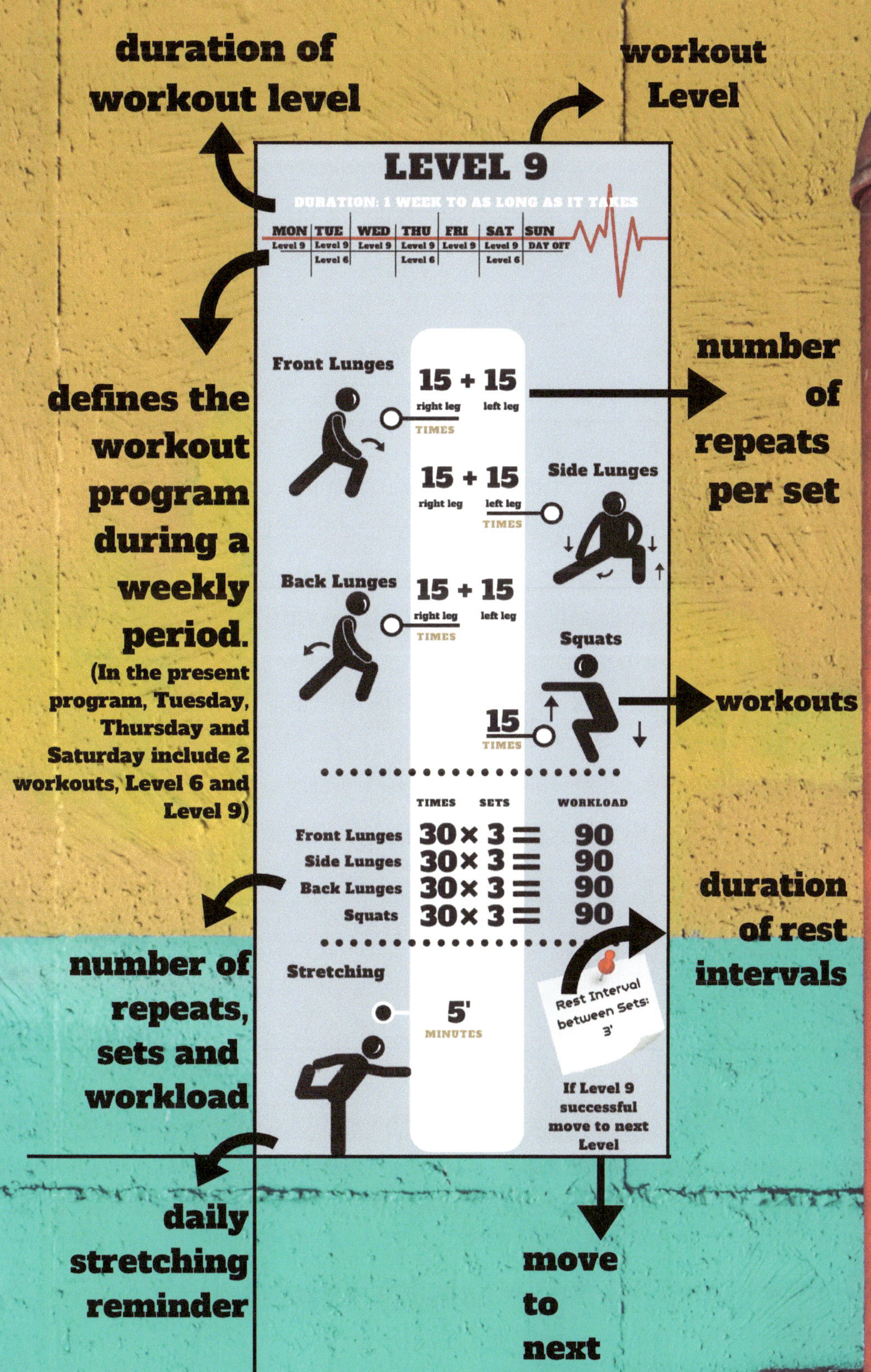

<u>Tips for LEVEL 1-6 Workouts</u>

- Always do stretching and warm-ups before workouts,
- keep a steady tempo during the workout,
- breathe in at the eccentric (easy) phase of the workout, breathe out at the concentric (difficult) phase of it.

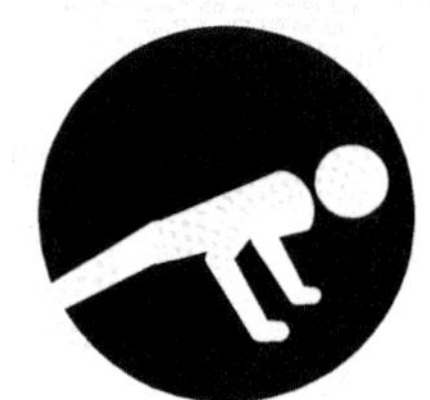

Push – ups

- One of the most challenging workouts. It requires the engagement of many muscles during workout (abdominals, triceps, pectorals, deltoids) plus the understanding of the core stability and body movement. Apart from a body workout, push-up workouts can be a demanding mental challenge. It requires the full body and mind concentration for achieving the right result.
- Back and legs should be fully straight. The legs must not touch the ground. When legs are extended there is a 70-75% body weightpush instead of a 50-60% when there is a kneeling push-up.
- Raise and lower your body by using your arms.

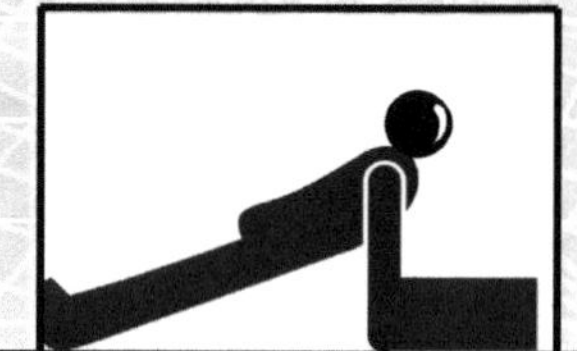

Triceps in Bench

- The hands should be placed on the edge of the bench. Elbows as close as possible to the body. Legs are stretched, resting on the heels.
- You lower yourself until your elbows form a 90° degree angle with a slow and controlled movement.
- Slowly return to starting position, by forcing on triceps.
- Elbows should not be widened during exercise.

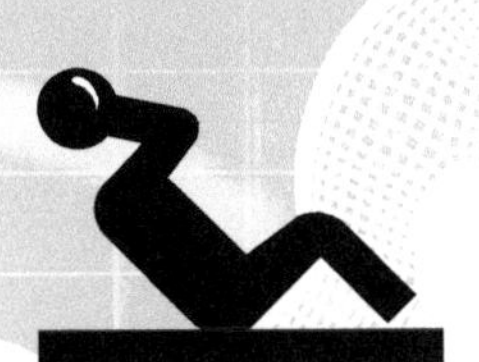

- The knees should bend at a 90° degree angle. Feet should be flat on the surface.
- For hands position there are two choices: either cross your arms over the chest or place your fingertips so that they barely touch your ears. You should never hold the head, as you can cause neck problems during workout.
- Make sure that your lumbar spine touches the surface the whole time during workout.
- The core should roll during the execution of the workout.
- At the beginning of the crunches workout, cervical spine should bend first, then thoracic spine follows and finally lumbar spine bends but without leaving contact with the surface.
- Nobody holds your feet, neither have you anchored them during sit-ups. If you do so, you reduce the workout of the abdominals and increase the workout of other muscles (iliopsoas, rectus fermoris).
- If lumbar spine is not touching the surface, or your feet are anchored during workout, there is a big possibility to increase the size of the iliopsoas muscle. Increase of iliopsoas muscle might cause increase of the lumbar lordosis.

Back 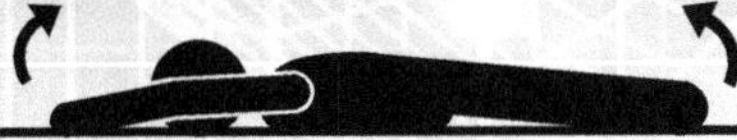 Extensions

- You should do a back extension slowly and under control. Rapid movements should be avoided, as they might lead to an injury.
- We never stretch the whole core during workout.
- The neck should bend during workout.
- Abdominals should always touch the surface.

LEVEL 1

DURATION: 1 DAY TO AS LONG AS IT TAKES

MON	TUE	WED	THU	FRI	SAT	SUN
Level 1	Level 1	Level 1	Level 1	Level 1	Level 1	Level 1

Push-ups

10 TIMES

Crunches

10 TIMES

Triceps in Bench

10 TIMES

Back Extensions

10 TIMES

	TIMES	SETS		WORKLOAD
Push-ups	10 × 1	=		10
Triceps in Bench	10 × 1	=		10
Crunches	10 × 1	=		10
Back Extensions	10 × 1	=		10

Stretching

5' MINUTES

Rest Interval between Sets: FREE

If Level 1 successful move to next Level

LEVEL 2

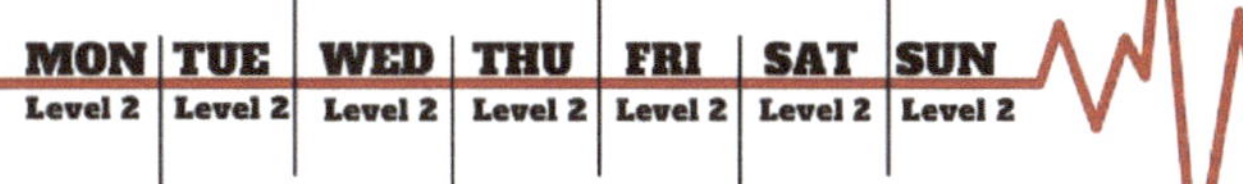

LEVEL 2

DURATION: 1 WEEK TO AS LONG AS IT TAKES

MON	TUE	WED	THU	FRI	SAT	SUN
Level 2	Level 2	Level 2	Level 2	Level 2	Level 2	Level 2

Push-ups

10 TIMES

Triceps in Bench

10 TIMES

Crunches

10 TIMES

Back Extensions

10 TIMES

	TIMES	SETS	WORKLOAD
Push-ups	10 × 5	=	50
Triceps in Bench	10 × 5	=	50
Crunches	10 × 5	=	50
Back Extensions	10 × 5	=	50

Stretching

5' MINUTES

Rest Interval between Sets: FREE

If Level 2 successful move to next Level

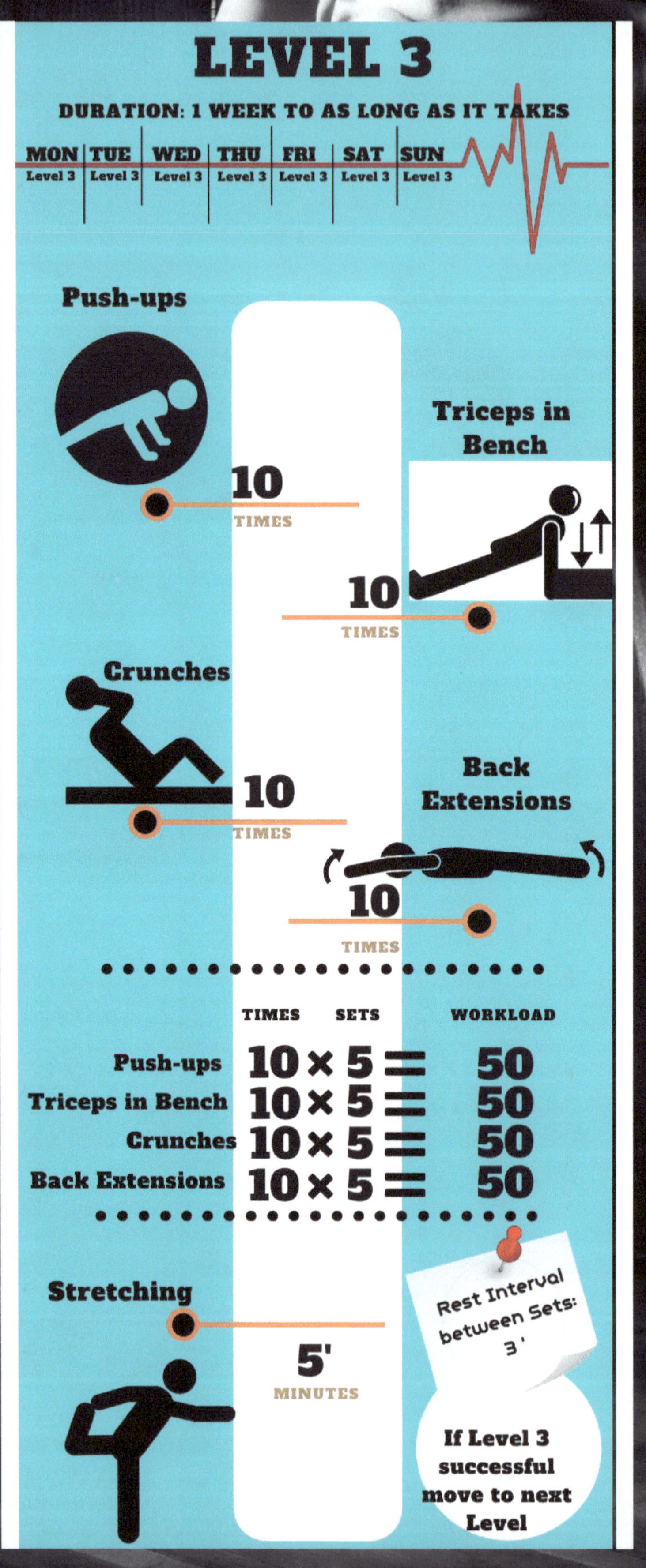

LEVEL 3
DURATION: 1 WEEK TO AS LONG AS IT TAKES
MON | TUE | WED | THU | FRI | SAT | SUN
Level 3 | Level 3 | Level 3 | Level 3 | Level 3 | Level 3 | Level 3
Push-ups
10 TIMES
Triceps in Bench
10 TIMES
Crunches
10 TIMES
Back Extensions
10 TIMES
TIMES   SETS   WORKLOAD
Push-ups   10 × 5 = 50
Triceps in Bench 10 × 5 = 50
Crunches   10 × 5 = 50
Back Extensions   10 × 5 = 50
Stretching
5' MINUTES
Rest Interval between Sets: 3'
If Level 3 successful move to next Level

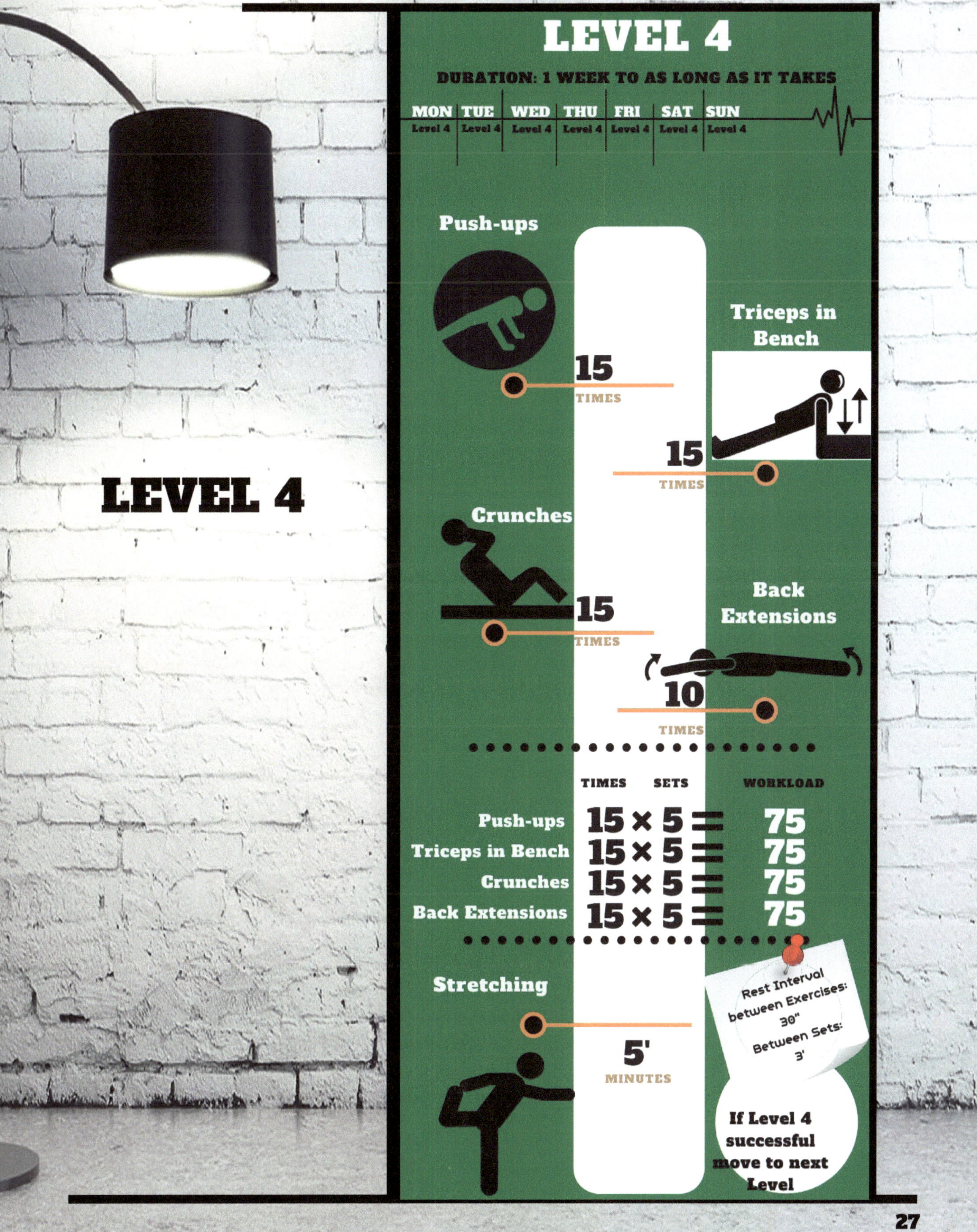

LEVEL 4
DURATION: 1 WEEK TO AS LONG AS IT TAKES
MON TUE WED THU FRI SAT SUN
Level 4 Level 4 Level 4 Level 4 Level 4 Level 4 Level 4
Push-ups
15 TIMES
Triceps in Bench
15 TIMES
Crunches
15 TIMES
Back Extensions
10 TIMES
TIMES   SETS   WORKLOAD
Push-ups   15 × 5 = 75
Triceps in Bench 15 × 5 = 75
Crunches   15 × 5 = 75
Back Extensions 15 × 5 = 75
Stretching
5' MINUTES
Rest Interval between Exercises: 30"
Between Sets: 3'
If Level 4 successful move to next Level
LEVEL 4

LEVEL 5

DURATION: 1 WEEK TO AS LONG AS IT TAKES

MON	TUE	WED	THU	FRI	SAT	SUN
Level 5	Level 5	Level 5	Level 5	Level 5	Level 5	Level 5

Push-ups

20 TIMES

Triceps in Bench

20 TIMES

Crunches

20 TIMES

Back Extensions

20 TIMES

	TIMES	SETS	WORKLOAD
Push-ups	20 × 5 =		100
Triceps in Bench	20 × 5 =		100
Crunches	20 × 5 =		100
Back Extensions	20 × 5 =		100

Stretching

5' MINUTES

Rest Interval between Exercises: 30"
Between Sets: 2'

If Level 5 successful move to next Level

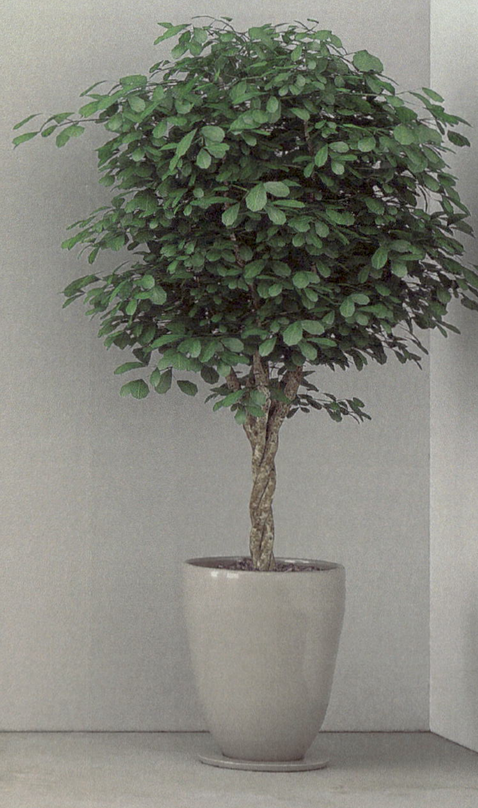

LEVEL 6

LEVEL 6
DURATION: 1 WEEK TO AS LONG AS IT TAKES
MON TUE WED THU FRI SAT SUN
Level 6 Level 6 Level 6 Level 6 Level 6 Level 6 Level 6
Push-ups
20 TIMES
Triceps in Bench
20 TIMES
Crunches
20 TIMES
Back Extensions
20 TIMES
TIMES SETS WORKLOAD
Push-ups 20 × 5 = 100
Triceps in Bench 20 × 5 = 100
Crunches 20 × 5 = 100
Back Extensions 20 × 5 = 100
Stretching
5' MINUTES
No Rest Interval between Exercises
Rest Interval Between Sets: 1'
If Level 5 successful move to next Level

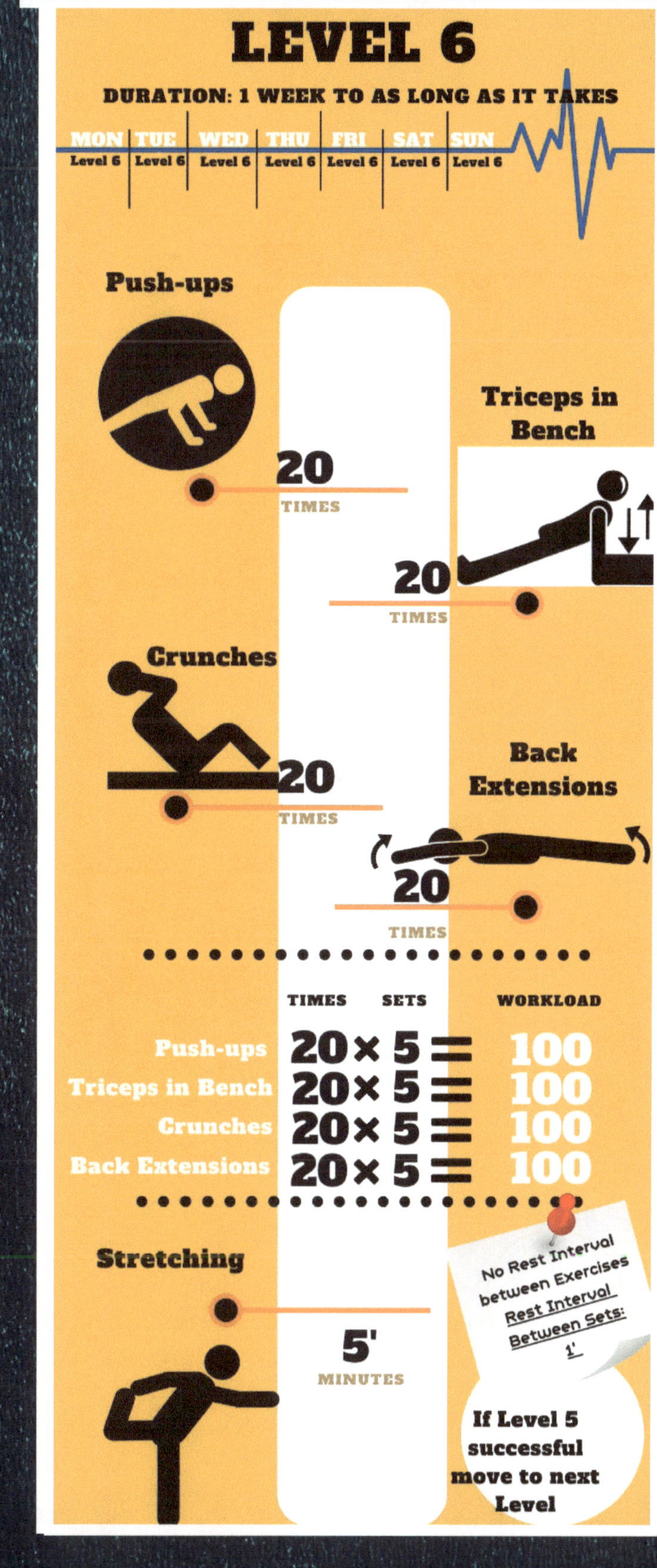

Part 2
LEVELS 7-11

Workouts for lower body muscles

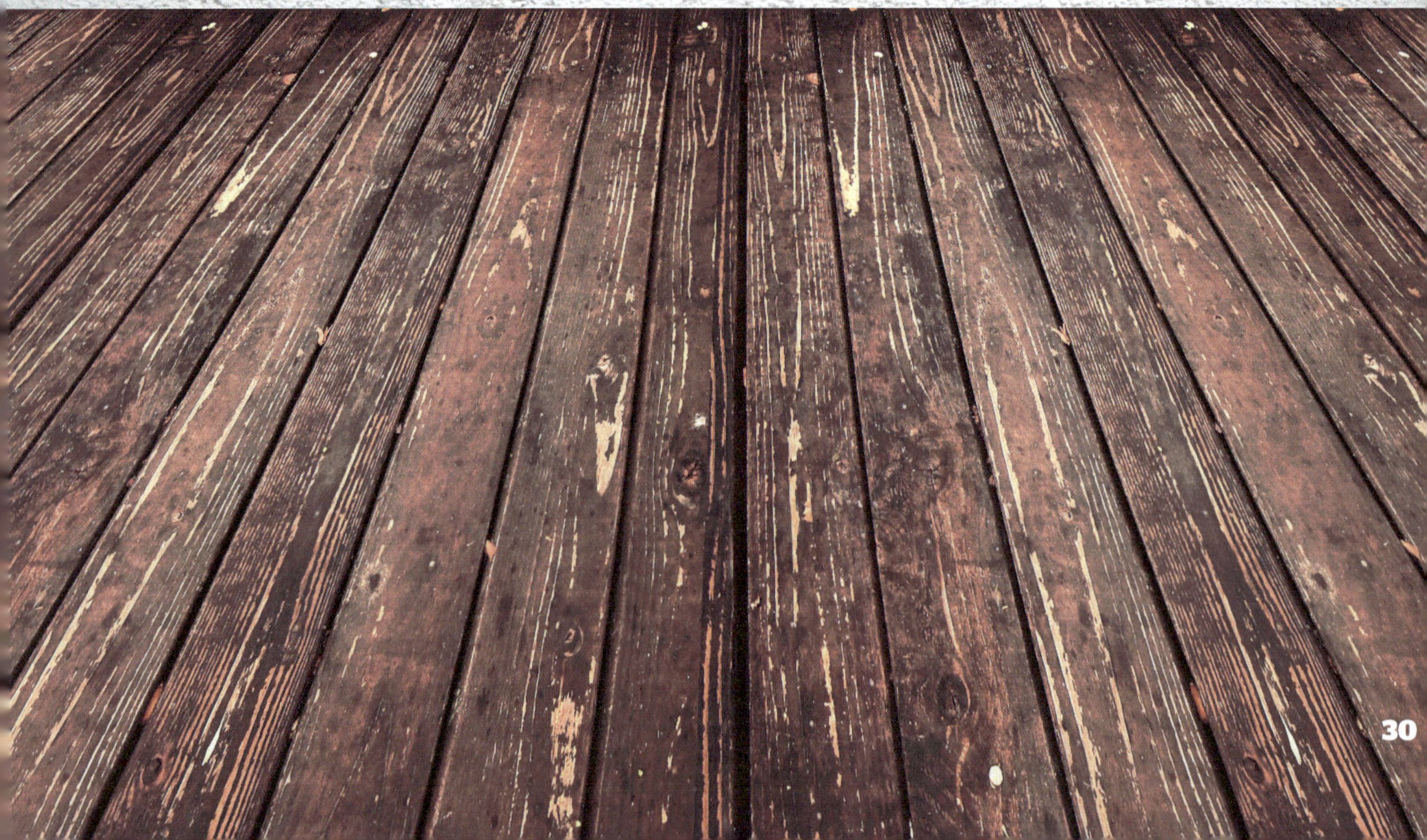

<u>Tips for **LEVEL 7-11 Workouts**</u>

Program for 7-11 Workouts includes also the LEVEL 6 Workouts three (3) times a week
(check Program in 7-11 Workout sheets).

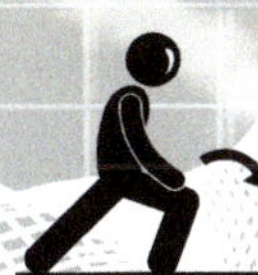

<u>Front Lunges</u>

- Place your arms on your waist; take a step forward and lunge.
- You must hold your front knee in line with your hip and ankle and lower your back knee toward the floor without touching it (if is really hard for you, you can hold on to the knee area until you get strong enough to do it without help).
- It is ok for the knees to extend beyond the toes during lunges workout. However, if you have a knee problem or pain in the knee area, it would be wise not to extend further than toes.
- Avoid arching your back.
- Return to original position and repeat.

<u>Back Lunges</u>

- Same starting position with Front Lunges, but instead of steping forward, you take a step to the back and lunge. Same principles with Front Lunges. Return to original position and repeat.

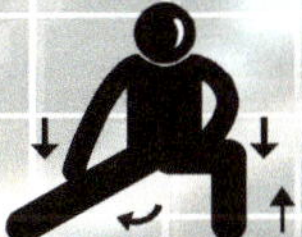

<u>Side Lunges</u>

- Same strarting position with Front Lunges, but instead of steping forward, you take a step to the side and slide with one leg stretched. Kneel down with the other foot. Return to original position and repeat.

<u>Squats</u>

- Squats are increasing the strength of lower body muscles and core.
- The feet should be placed apart on shoulder-width. The eyes are looking in front. Cross your arms in chest or hold your arms out in front at shoulder height.
- Keep your back as straight as you can and avoid arching.
- From standing position you lower the hips. At the bottom of the exercise you pause for a moment and then strongly stand back up to the starting position. It will be easier for you if you push through the outer edges of your feet. Repeat.

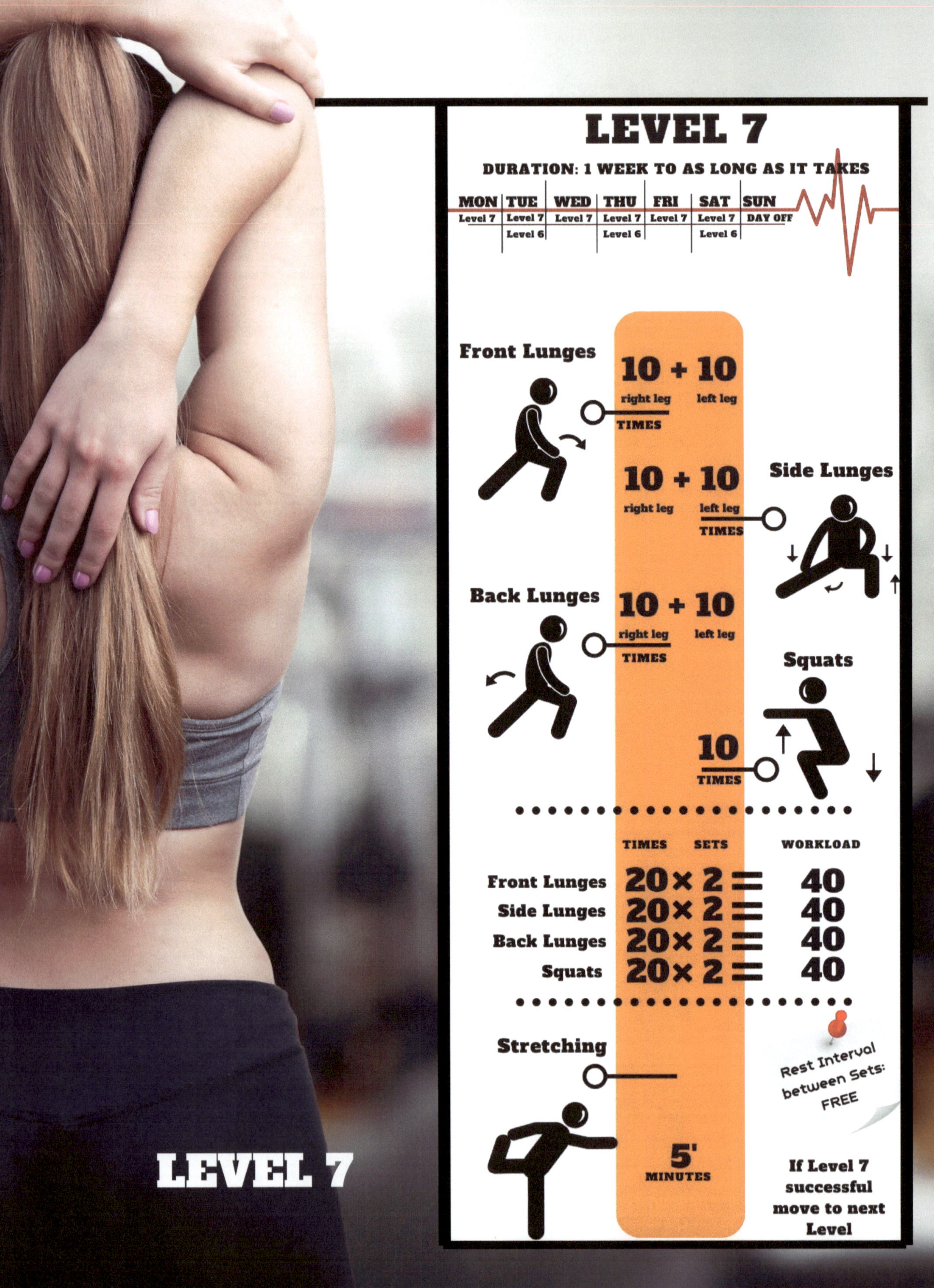

LEVEL 7

DURATION: 1 WEEK TO AS LONG AS IT TAKES

MON | TUE | WED | THU | FRI | SAT | SUN
Level 7 | Level 7 | Level 7 | Level 7 | Level 7 | Level 7 | DAY OFF
| Level 6 | | Level 6 | | Level 6 |

Front Lunges
10 + 10
right leg   left leg
TIMES

10 + 10
right leg   left leg
TIMES

Side Lunges

Back Lunges
10 + 10
right leg   left leg
TIMES

Squats
10
TIMES

TIMES   SETS   WORKLOAD
Front Lunges   20 × 2 = 40
Side Lunges   20 × 2 = 40
Back Lunges   20 × 2 = 40
Squats   20 × 2 = 40

Stretching
5'
MINUTES

Rest Interval between Sets: FREE

If Level 7 successful move to next Level

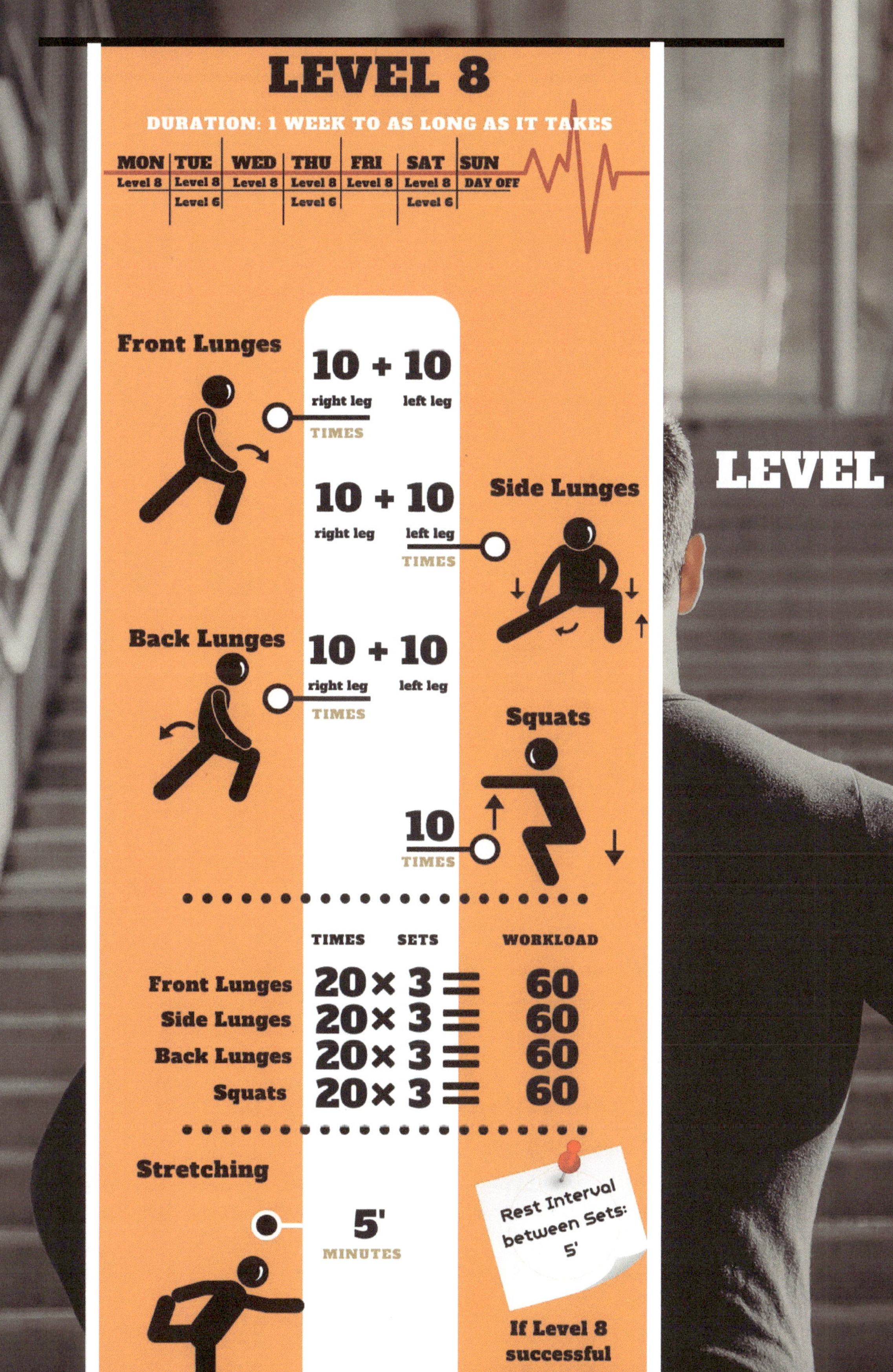

LEVEL 8
DURATION: 1 WEEK TO AS LONG AS IT TAKES
MON TUE WED THU FRI SAT SUN
Level 8 Level 8 Level 8 Level 8 Level 8 Level 8 DAY OFF
Level 6 Level 6 Level 6
Front Lunges
10 + 10
right leg left leg
TIMES
10 + 10
right leg left leg
TIMES
Side Lunges
Back Lunges
10 + 10
right leg left leg
TIMES
Squats
10
TIMES
TIMES SETS WORKLOAD
Front Lunges 20 × 3 = 60
Side Lunges 20 × 3 = 60
Back Lunges 20 × 3 = 60
Squats 20 × 3 = 60
Stretching
5'
MINUTES
Rest Interval between Sets: 5'
If Level 8 successful move to next Level

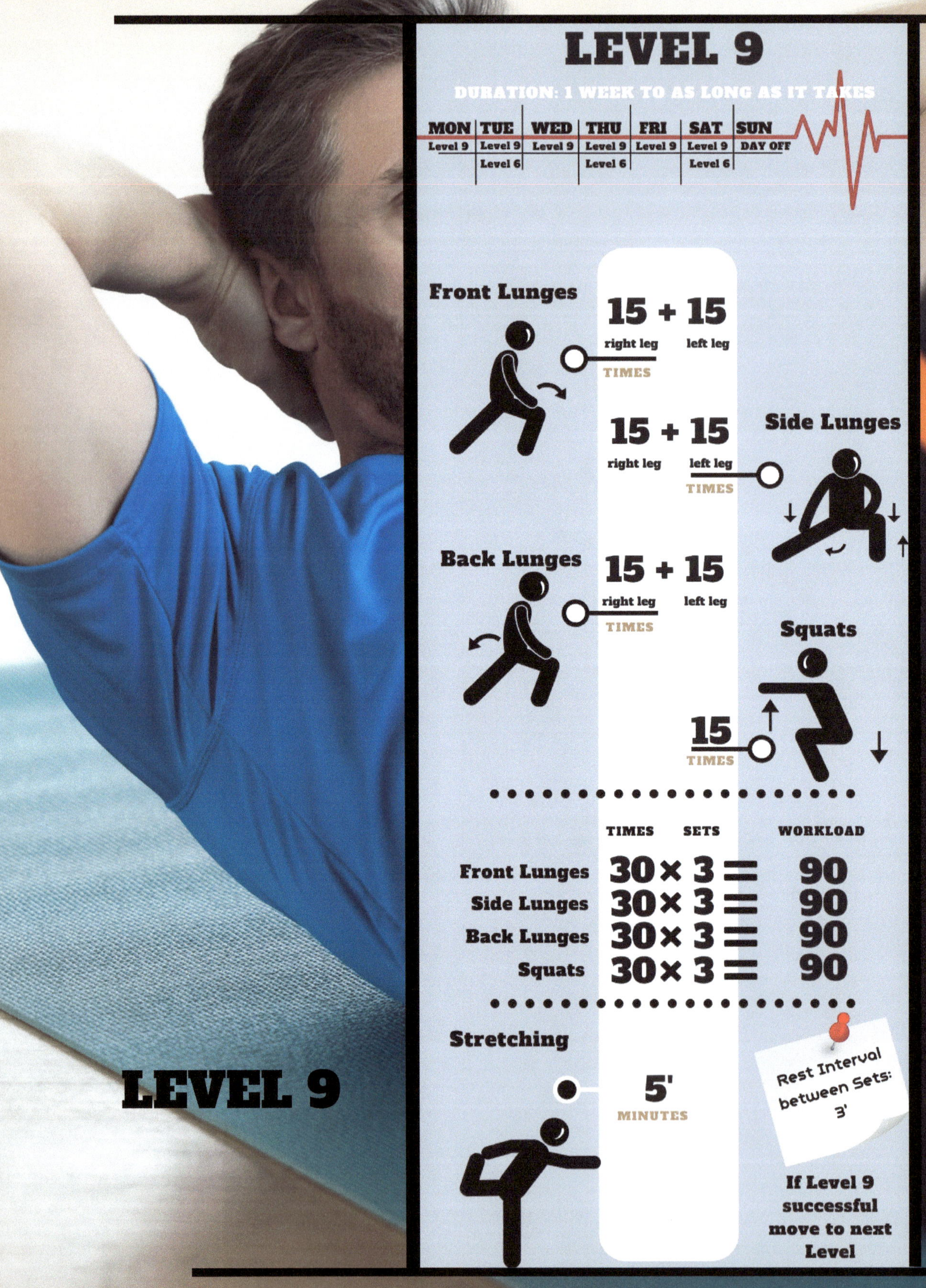

LEVEL 9
DURATION: 1 WEEK TO AS LONG AS IT TAKES
MON Level 9
TUE Level 9 Level 6
WED Level 9
THU Level 9 Level 6
FRI Level 9
SAT Level 9 Level 6
SUN DAY OFF
Front Lunges
15 + 15
right leg   left leg
TIMES
15 + 15
right leg   left leg
TIMES
Side Lunges
Back Lunges
15 + 15
right leg   left leg
TIMES
Squats
15
TIMES
TIMES   SETS   WORKLOAD
Front Lunges   30 × 3 = 90
Side Lunges   30 × 3 = 90
Back Lunges   30 × 3 = 90
Squats   30 × 3 = 90
Stretching
5'
MINUTES
Rest Interval between Sets: 3'
If Level 9 successful move to next Level

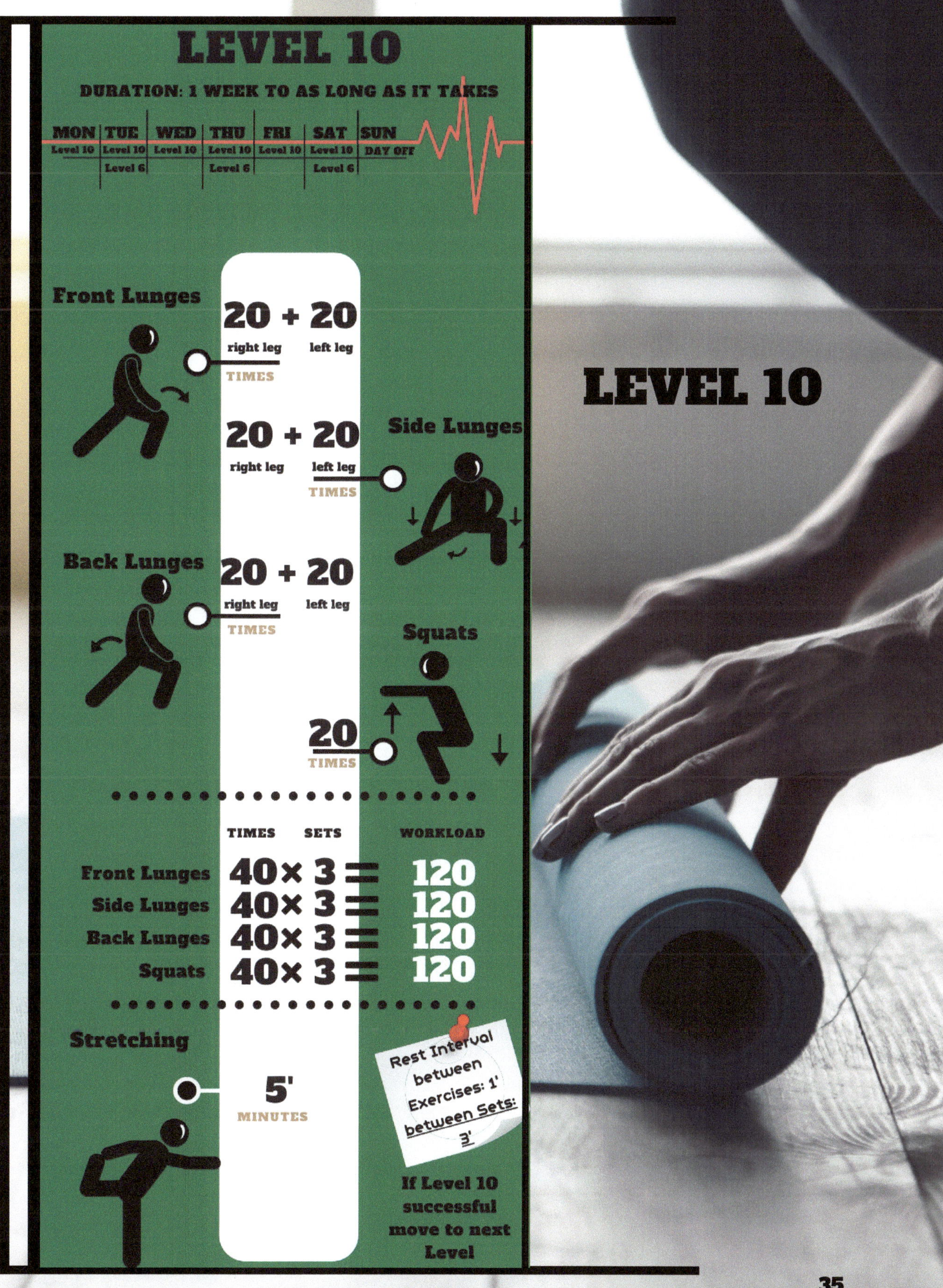
LEVEL 10
DURATION: 1 WEEK TO AS LONG AS IT TAKES
MON TUE WED THU FRI SAT SUN
Level 10 Level 10 Level 10 Level 10 Level 10 Level 10 DAY OFF
Level 6 Level 6 Level 6
Front Lunges
20 + 20
right leg left leg
TIMES
20 + 20
right leg left leg
TIMES
Side Lunges
Back Lunges
20 + 20
right leg left leg
TIMES
Squats
20
TIMES
TIMES SETS WORKLOAD
Front Lunges 40 × 3 = 120
Side Lunges 40 × 3 = 120
Back Lunges 40 × 3 = 120
Squats 40 × 3 = 120
Stretching
5'
MINUTES
Rest Interval between Exercises: 1'
between Sets: 3'
If Level 10 successful move to next Level
LEVEL 10

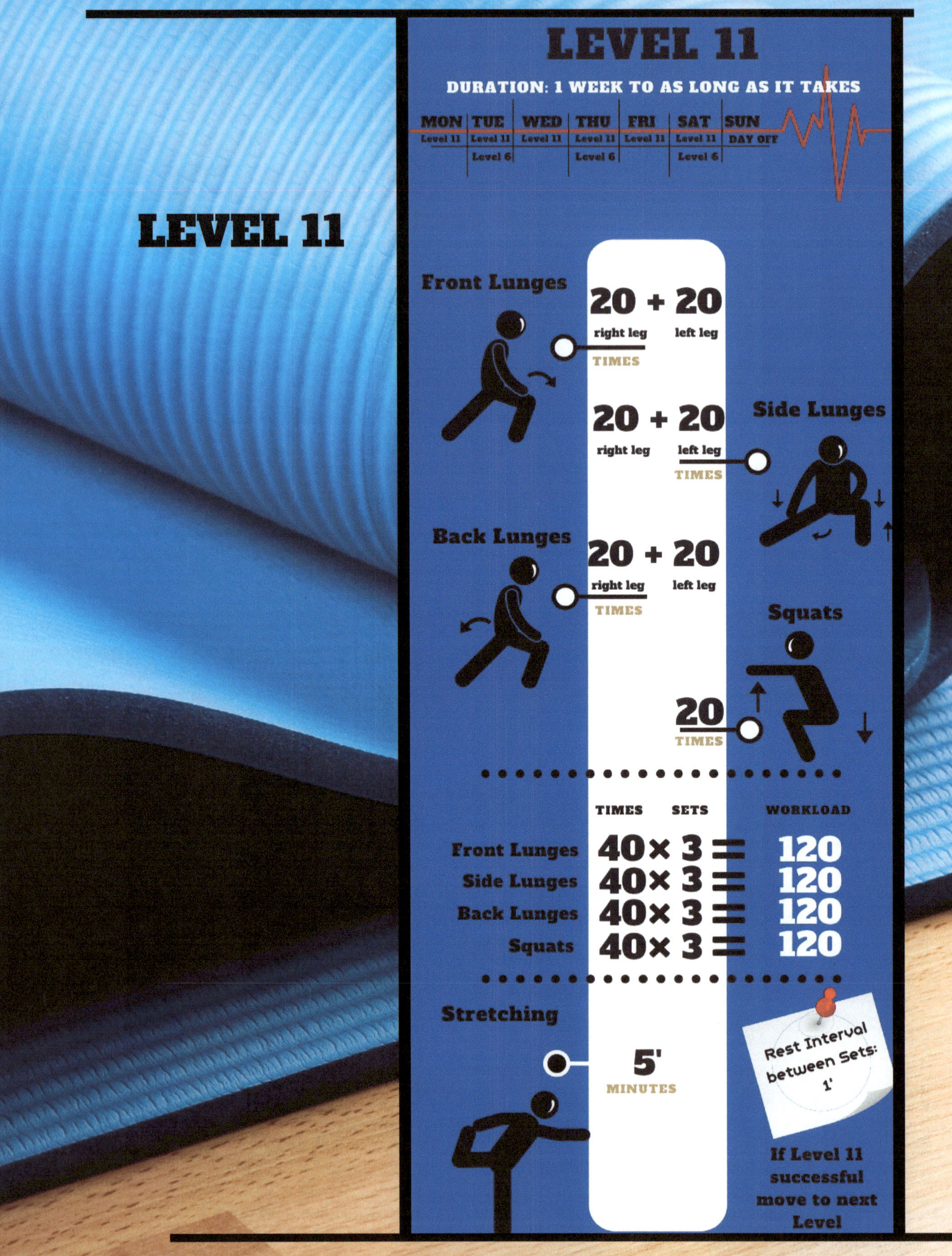

LEVEL 11
DURATION: 1 WEEK TO AS LONG AS IT TAKES
MON Level 11
TUE Level 11 / Level 6
WED Level 11
THU Level 11 / Level 6
FRI Level 11
SAT Level 11 / Level 6
SUN DAY OFF
Front Lunges
20 + 20
right leg   left leg
TIMES
20 + 20
right leg   left leg
TIMES
Side Lunges
Back Lunges
20 + 20
right leg   left leg
TIMES
Squats
20
TIMES
TIMES   SETS   WORKLOAD
Front Lunges   40 × 3   120
Side Lunges   40 × 3   120
Back Lunges   40 × 3   120
Squats   40 × 3   120
Stretching
5'
MINUTES
Rest Interval between Sets: 1'
If Level 11 successful move to next Level

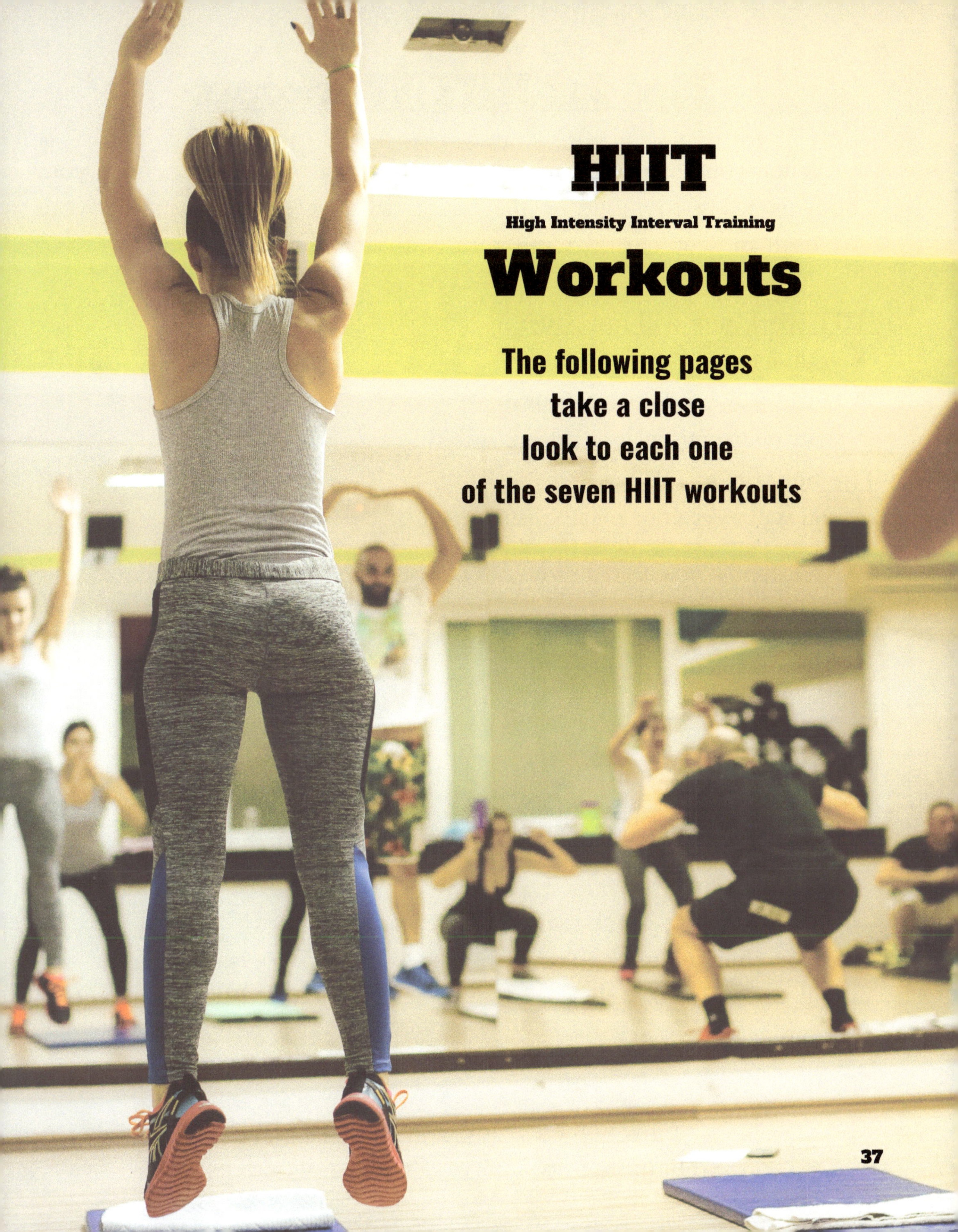

HIIT
High Intensity Interval Training
Workouts
The following pages
take a close
look to each one
of the seven HIIT workouts

Tips for HIIT Workouts

When you have completed the workout goals of LEVELS 7–11, your body is ready to move to the next challenge. You have built your strength and you have worked with your flexibility.

HIIT workouts will improve:
- your aerobic metabolism,
- your cardio–respiratory fitness,
- your neuromuscular adaption.

The benefits of HIIT:
- you will reset your metabolism,
- it will help you burn major fat,
- it will Improve your endurance,
- body will continue burning calories long after the end of the HIIT workouts.

Tips:
- **d**o not forget stretching (it will help muscles to get ready for the upcoming workouts and protect you from injuries),
- you might need to wear a pair of sport shoes for the HIIT workouts,
- breathe normally,
- do not forget to check the Heart Rate Zones,
- if you feel uncomfortable at any part of the workouts, you should stop and ask advise by a doctor for the type of workouts you should choose in order to exercise.

Now you are ready to work with HIIT
(High Intensity Interval Training) workouts.

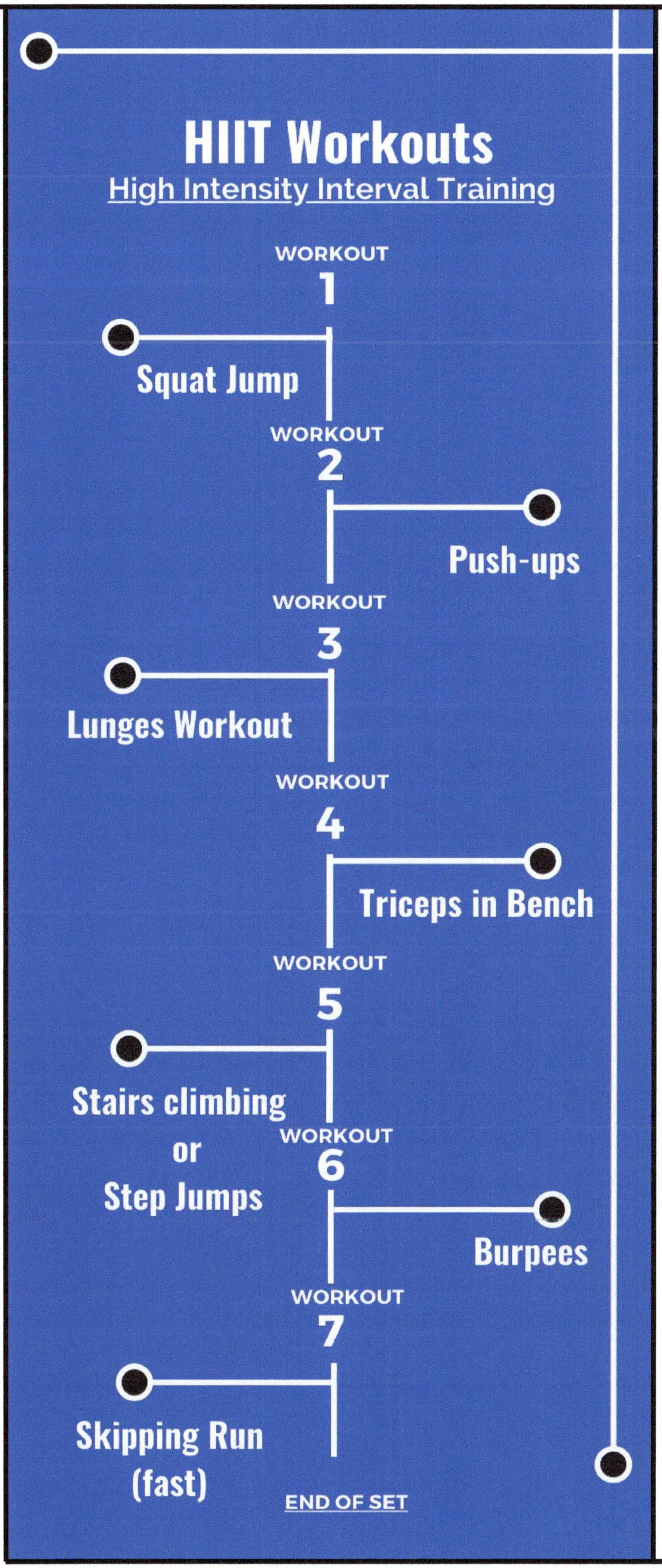

HIIT Workouts
High Intensity Interval Training

WORKOUT
1

Squat Jump

WORKOUT
2

Push-ups

WORKOUT
3

Lunges Workout

WORKOUT
4

Triceps in Bench

WORKOUT
5

Stairs climbing
or
Step Jumps

WORKOUT
6

Burpees

WORKOUT
7

Skipping Run
(fast)

END OF SET

Basic Rules for HIIT Workouts:

Perform workouts with any order you like. Try to select different muscle groups when changing workouts.

When HRMax during interval reaches below 50%, you can start again the workouts.

For better results, you should follow the planned HIIT program, regarding time, interval, Heart Rate and repetitions.

1. Squat Jump

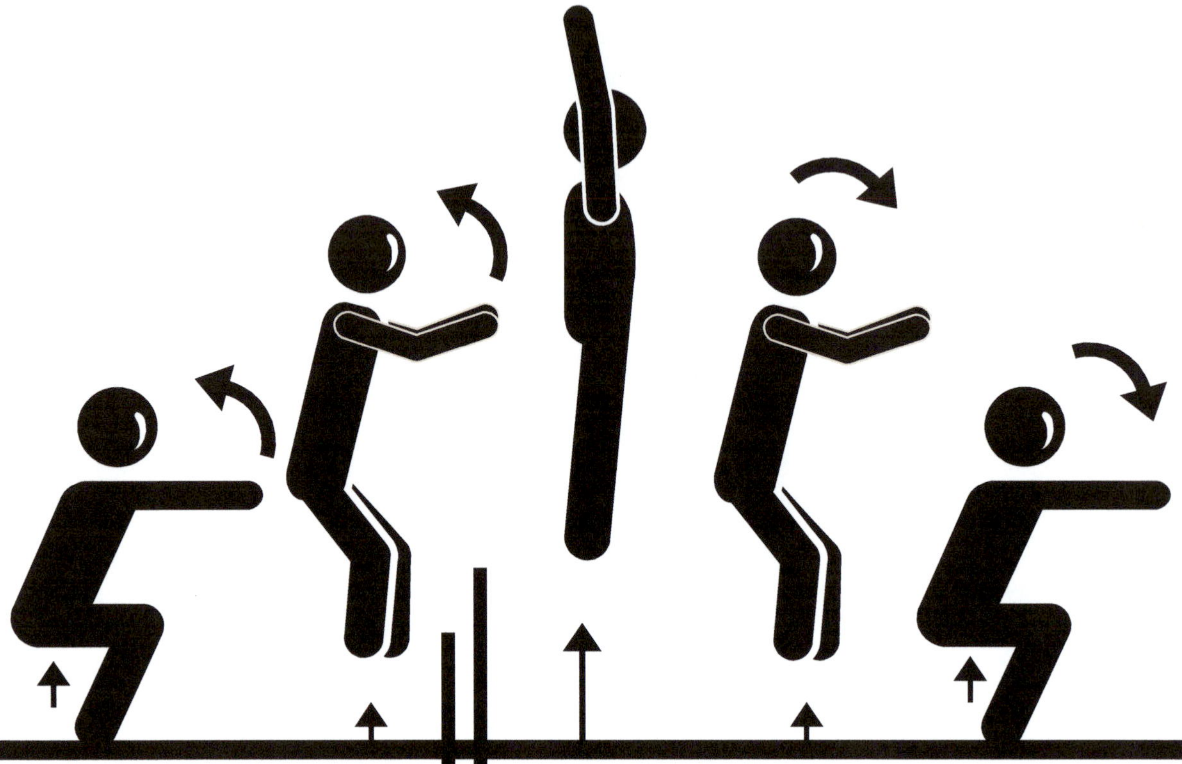

Tips.

1. Keep your back as straight as you can and avoid arching.

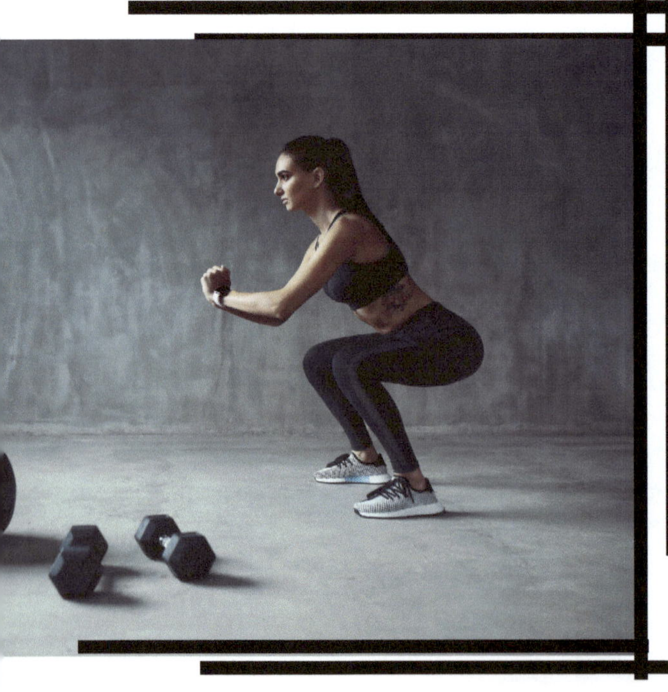

2. The feet should be placed apart on shoulder-width. The eyes are looking in front. Cross your arms in chest or hold your arms out in front at shoulder height.

3. From standing position you lower the hips. Lower down until your thighs are parallel to the floor. Press your feet down and jump as high as you can. Move your hands above your head for reaching the highest point possible.

4. Just as you land, allow knees to bend for 45° degrees, drop back down for a squat and jump again.

5. It will be easier for you if you push through the outer edges of your feet.

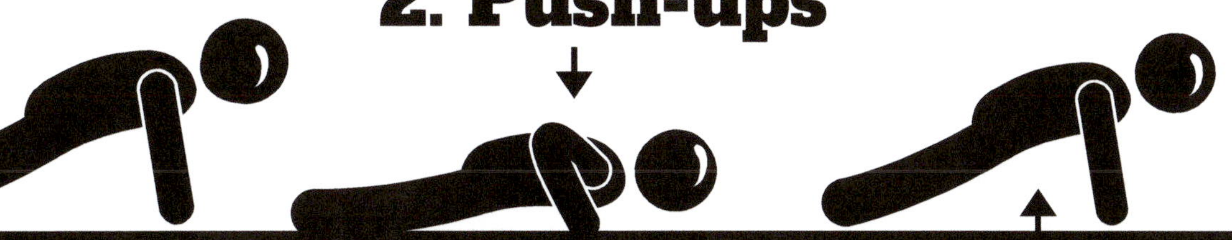

2. Push-ups

Tips.

1. When legs are extended there is a 70–75 % body weightpush. Instead there is a 50% of body weightpush for the kneeling push-up.

2. Pushups engage the workout of many muscles:
- abdominals,
- triceps,
- pectorals (chest muscles),
- deltoids (shoulder muscles),
- serratus anterior (wing muscles),
- plus the understanding of the core stability and body movement.

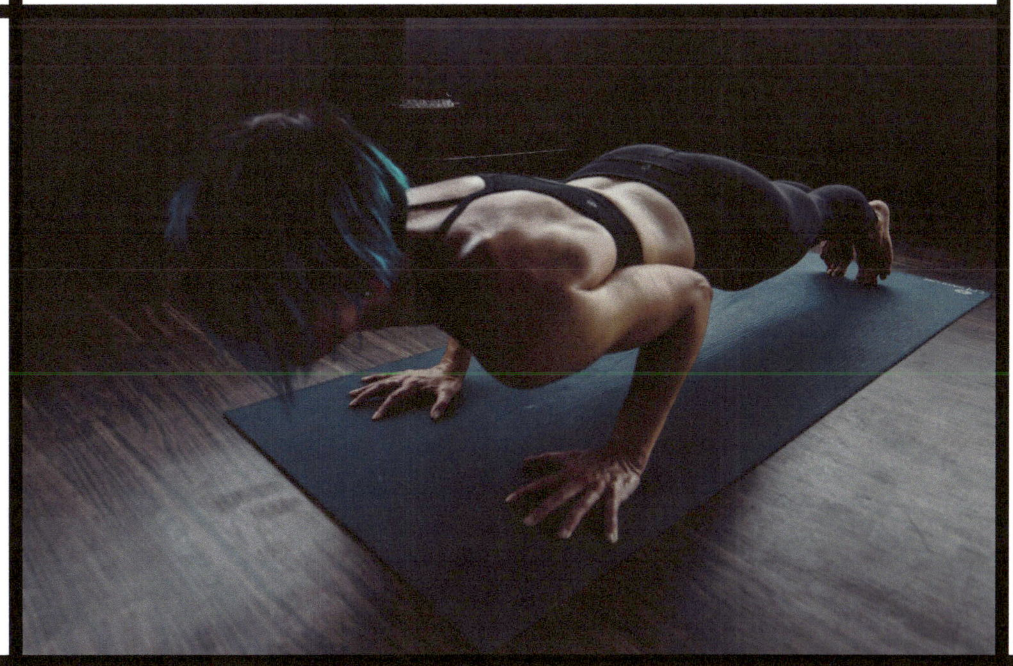

3. Lunges Workout

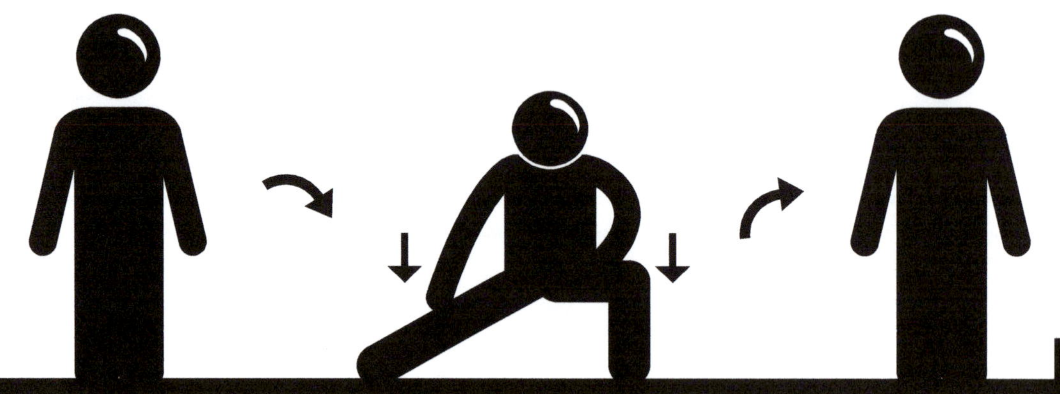

Tips.

1. Use different types of lunges (front, back, side) when changing sets.

2. It is ok for the knees to extend beyond the toes during lunges workout. However, if you have a knee problem or pain in the knee area, it would be wise not to extend further than toes.

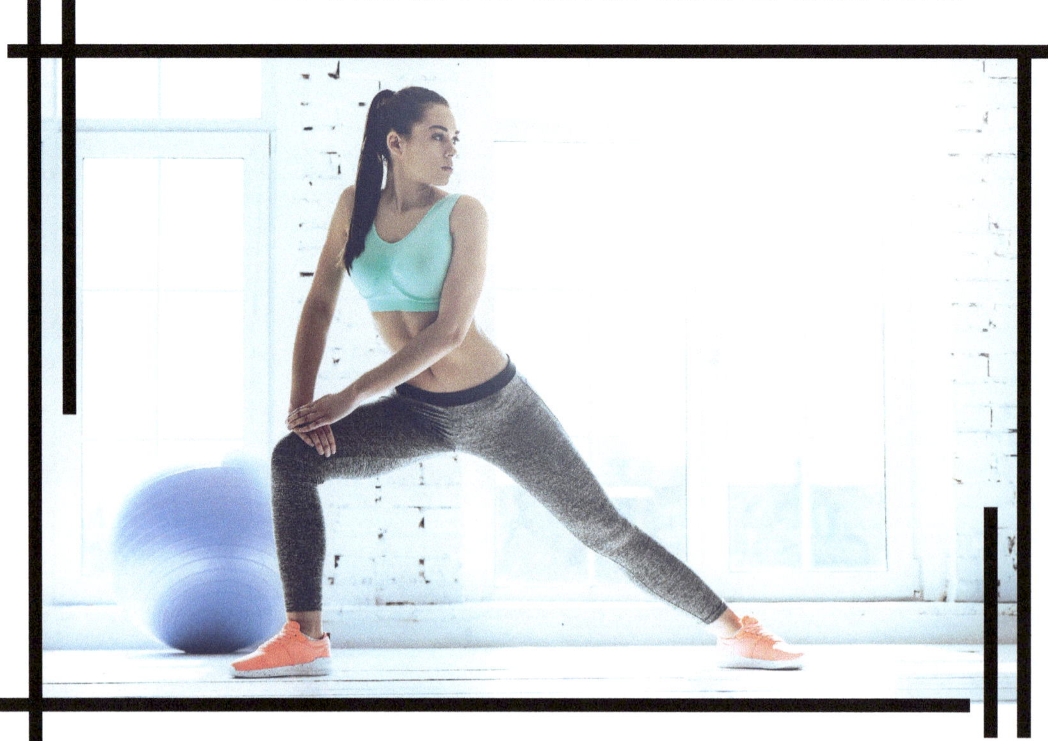

4. Triceps in Bench

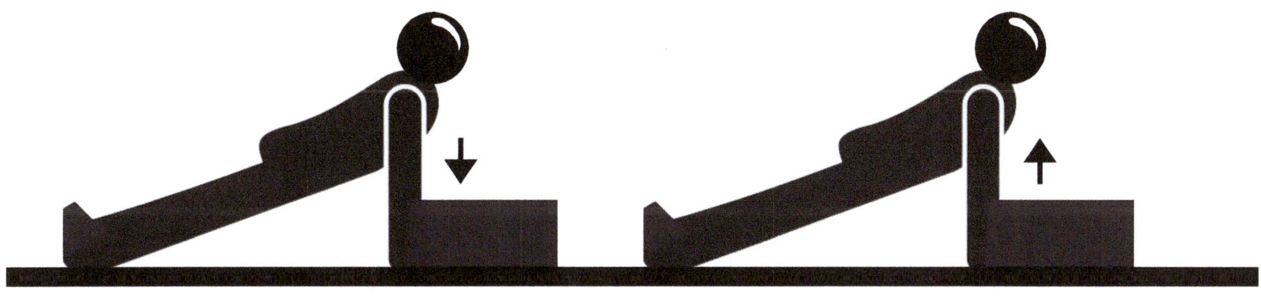

Tips.

1. The wrists get all the pressure during triceps workout. Before starting the workout, you should warm-up your wrists.

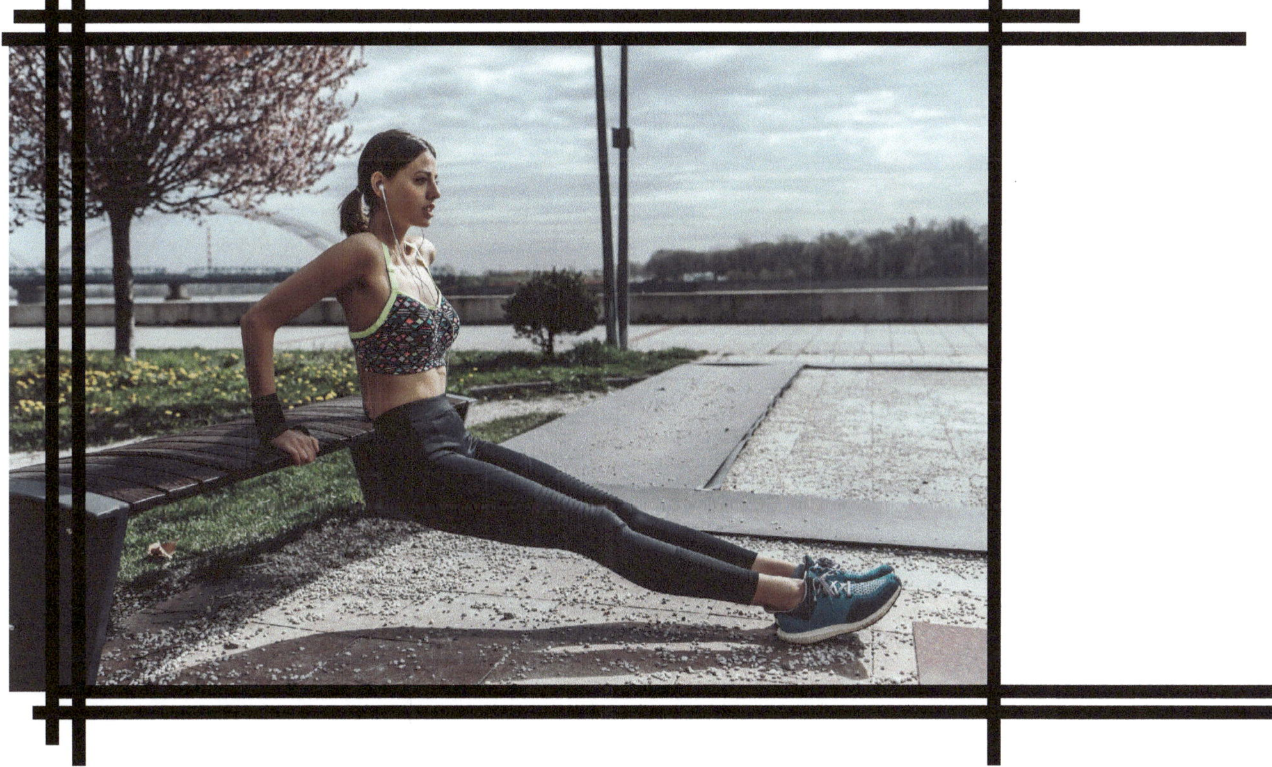

5. Stair Climbing

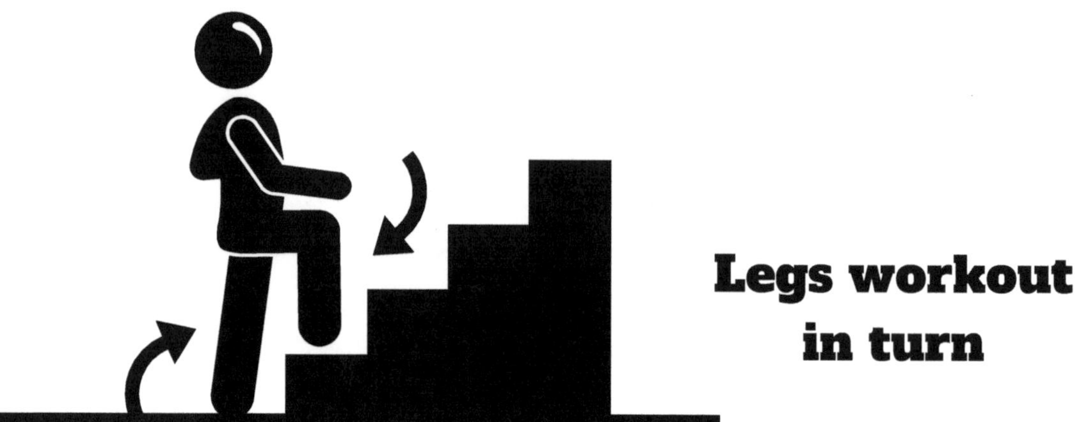

**Legs workout
in turn**

Or

5. Step Jumps

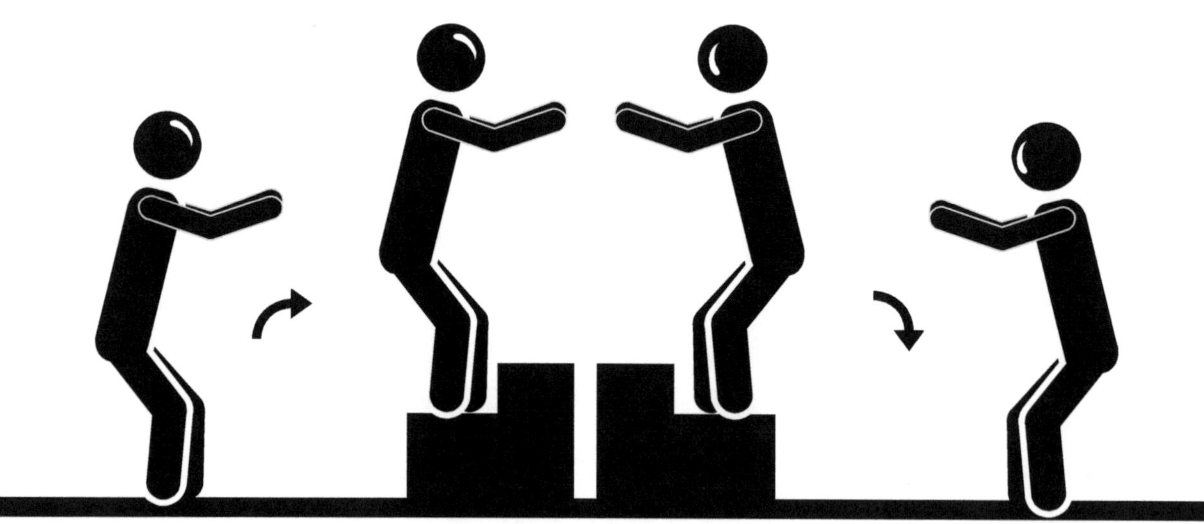

Keep a steady tempo during workouts!

6. Skipping Run (fast)

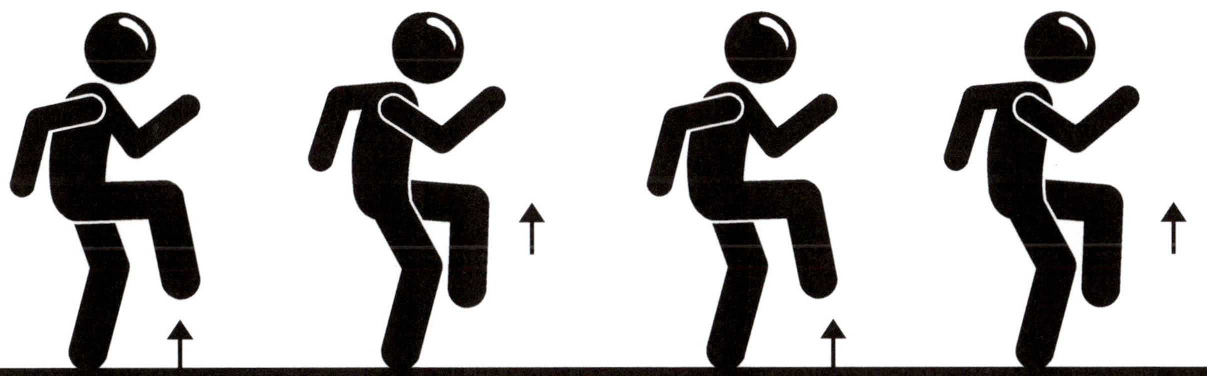

1. Perform skipping run in a fast tempo.

2. Bend your hands in a 90° degree angle.

Tips.

3. Perform forefoot running.

4. Lift your knees quite high during skipping run.

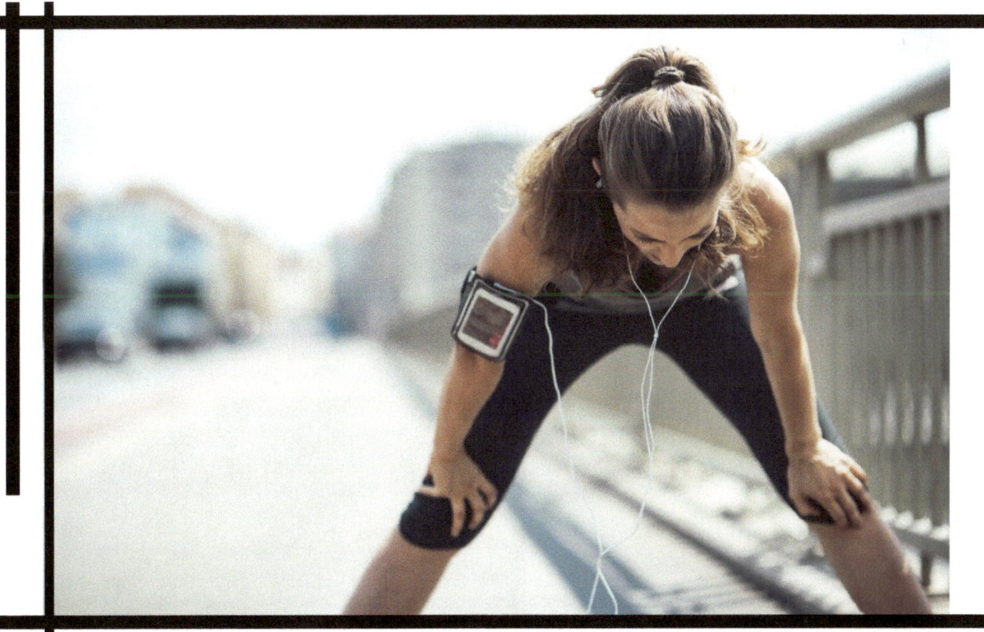

7. Burpees

Tips.

1. Start from standing position.

2. Move to squat position with hands placed on the ground.

3. Kick your feet back (plank position/ arms extended).

4. Quick return into squat position.

5. Steady position and jump.

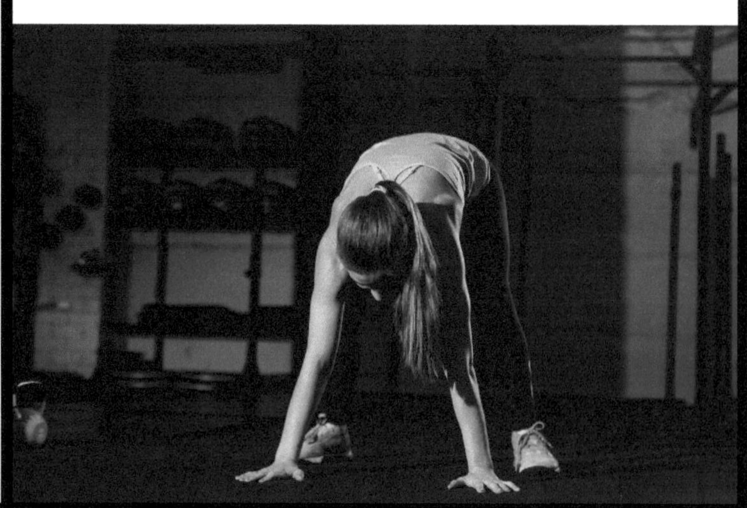

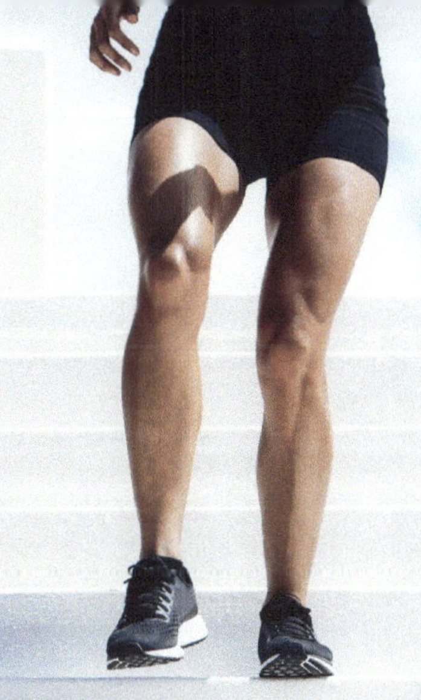

You will use the same seven (7) workouts. What varies is the repetitions of the workouts and the intervals from set to set!

You can use the HIIT workouts on a three different ways exercise system:

1. HIIT WORKOUT 1
2. HIIT WORKOUT 2
3. HIIT WORKOUT 3

HIIT WORKOUTS

7. Burpees

6. Skipping Run (Fast)

5. Stair Climbing or Step Jumps

4. Triceps in Bench

3. Lunges

2. Push-ups

1. Squat Jump

HIIT WORKOUTS 1-2-3 Comparison

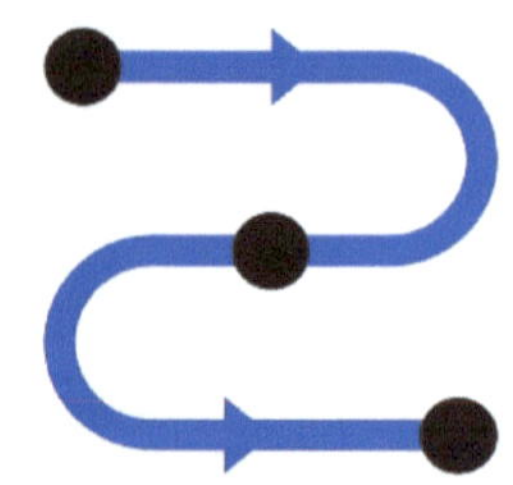

7 — Same workouts for each HIIT WORKOUT (1-2-3)

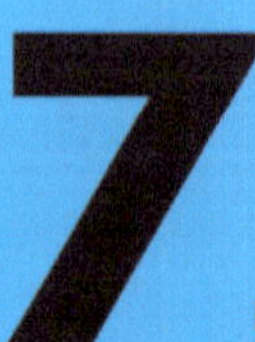

Squat Jump/Push-ups/Triceps in Bench/Lunges/Stair climbing or step jumps/ Burpees/Skipping run (fast)

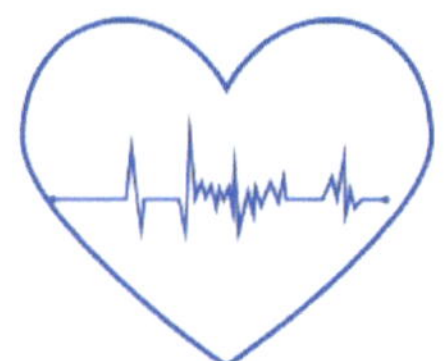

HR (HEART RATE) DURING ALL WORKOUTS SHOULD BE BETWEEN 70-84% HR MAX

This is the suggested **Heart Rate Zone** for a HIIT Workout.

WORKOUT REPETITIONS AND DURATION

HIIT workout 1:
Repetitions **without time** duration (8-10 REPS/WORKOUT)

HIIT workout 2:
Repetitions **with time** duration (6 REPS - SET DURATION: 3')

HIIT workout 3:
25" For each workout X 7 Workouts = 175" SET DURATION

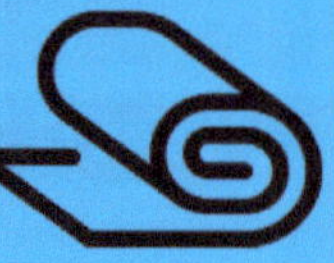

INTERVAL BETWEEN SETS: UNTIL HRMAX IS <50%.

HIIT WORKOUT 1 : INTERVAL UNTIL HR MAX **<50%**
HIIT WORKOUT 2: **6' (MIN)** INTERVAL AND UNTIL HR MAX **<50%**
HIIT WORKOUT 3: **7'(MIN)** INTERVAL UNTIL HR MAX **<50%**

4: Sets to complete each HIIT Workout

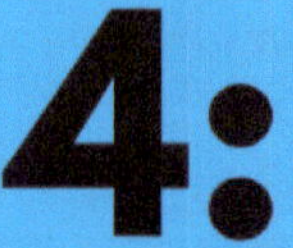

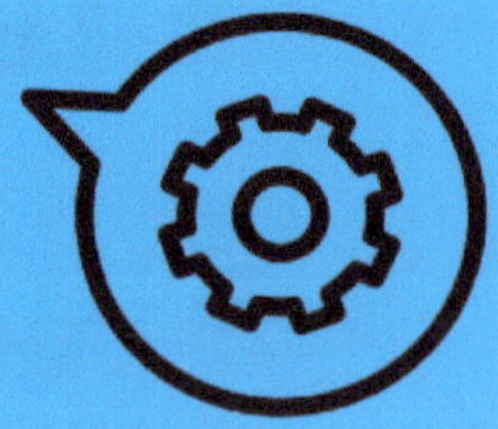

Before starting the HIIT Workouts, make sure that you have fully understood the exact technique of the mentioned workouts!

HIIT WORKOUTS 1

Do the 7 workouts with 8-10 repetitions on each workout, intensely executed.

Work in the 70-84% of the maximum Heart Rate.

Immediate transition from one workout to the other.

When you are finished with the total 7 workouts, 1 Set is completed.

Rest and start again the new set when HRmax is <50%.

For achieving HIIT Workout 1, you need to complete 4 Sets in total.

HIIT WORKOUTS 1

Number of workouts:	7	**Heart Rate Zone:**	70-84% HR max
Repetitions per set:	8-10	**Workouts Interval:**	None
Number of sets:	4	**Sets Interval:**	Until HR max is <50%

HOW TO WORK WITH HIIT WORKOUTS 1

There are 7 workouts

Squat Jump/Push-ups/Triceps in Bench/Lunges/Stairs climbing or step jumps/ Burpees/Skipping run (fast) are the seven workouts that you will need for HIIT Workouts 1.

Heart Rate Zone

For best working results, your Heart Rate Zone should be within the 70-84% of the Maximum Heart Rate (HR max).

Repetitions: 8-10

You should repeat 8-10 times each Workout on each SET. For begginers it is suggested to start from 8 repetitions and when they are ready to continue with 10 repetitions

Interval between Workouts

There are no intervals between the 7 workouts. You should rotate from one workout to the other without interval.

Number of Sets: 4

You should perform 4 sets for a successful HIIT Workouts 1.
7 Workouts = 1 Set
4 Sets = 1 HIIT

Interval between Sets

After you complete a Set of workouts (7) you can take a break. During the Interval, you regulary check your Heart Rate. When your Heart Rate is <50% of the HR max, you can continue with the next Set of HIIT Workouts.

Tips:
- you can rotate Lunges workouts (front/back/side lunges) during sets,
- the Heart Rate table will help you define your HRmax according to your age,
- if your Heart Rate Zone is higher than 70-84% of HRmax, reduce repetitions until you manage to get your Heart Rate to that Zone. Go back to the original repetitions when you feel ready again,
- interval between sets is really important. Do not start before your Heart Rate is <50% HRmax.

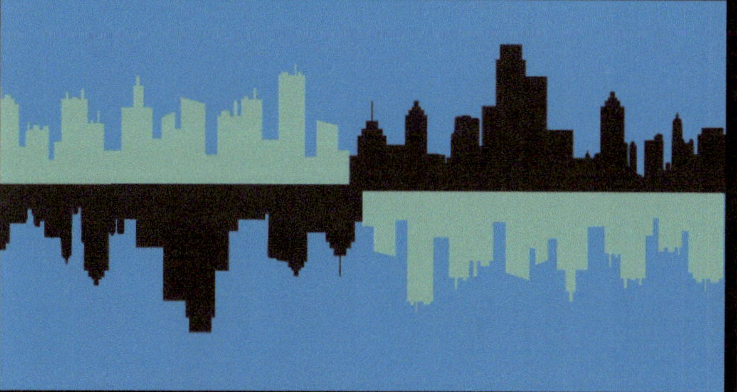

HIIT WORKOUTS 2

Number of workouts: 7	**Heart Rate Zone:** 70-84% of HR max
Repetitions per set: 6	**Workouts Interval:** None
Set Duration: 3'	**Sets Interval:** 6' and HR max is <50%
Number of sets: 4	**Purpose:** Perform as many workouts you can within 3' minutes time.

HOW TO WORK WITH HIIT WORKOUTS 2

There are 7 workouts

Squat Jump/Push-ups/Triceps in Bench/Lunges/Stair climbing or step jumps/ Burpees/Skipping run (fast) are the seven workouts that you will need for HIIT Workouts 2.

Repetitions: 6

You should repeat 6 times each Workout on each SET.

Set Duration: 3'

Duration of each Set is 3 minutes time (3'). You should perform as many workouts as you can in rotation during that period (remember: 6 repetitions per workout). Count the workouts on each set.

Number of Sets: 4

You should perform 4 sets for a successful HIIT Workouts 2.
3' min of workouts = 1 Set
4 Sets = HIIT Workouts 2

Heart Rate Zone

For best working results, your Heart Rate Zone should be within the 70-84% of the Maximum Heart Rate (HR max).

Interval between Workouts

There are no intervals between workouts. You should rotate from one workout to the other without interval for a period of 3 minutes (3') time.

Interval between Sets:6'

After you complete a Set (Set Duration = 3') you can take a break. During the interval, check regularly your Heart Rate. When six minutes (6') have passed and your Heart Rate is <50% of the HR max, you can continue with the next Set of HIIT Workouts.

Tips:
- use a timer to count the Set Duration (3'),
- rotate workouts every 6 repetitions / do as many workouts as you can,
- the Heart Rate Table will help you define your HRmax according to your age,
- if your Heart Rate Zone is higher than 70-84% of HRmax, reduce repetitions until you manage to get your Heart Rate to that Zone. Go back to the original repetitions when you feel ready again,
- interval between sets is really important. Do not start before your Heart Rate is <50% of HRmax.

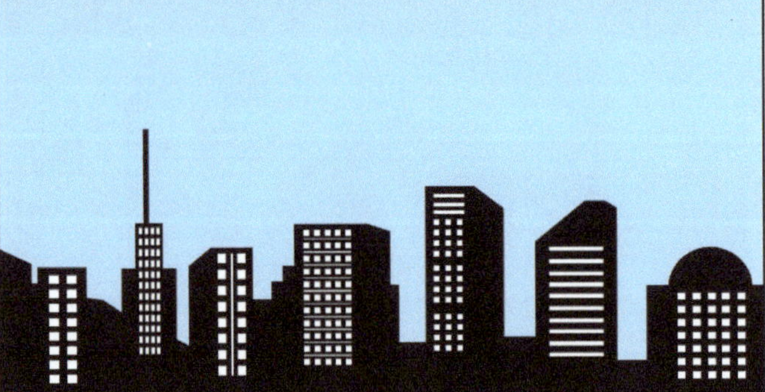

HIIT WORKOUTS 2

There are 6 repetitions on each workout, intensely executed.

Rotate the 7 workouts again and again until 3 minutes' period ends.

You should count the workouts executed so as to mark down your progress.

Work in the 70-84% of the maximum Heart Rate (HRmax).

Immediate transition from one workout to the other.

When a workout period of 3 minutes' ends, 1 Set is completed.

Rest for 6 minutes and check if your HRmax is <50%. If so, start again another set of workouts.

For achieving HIIT Workout 2, you need to complete 4 Sets in total.

"

HIIT WORKOUTS 3

Repetitions on each workout last 25'' seconds.

Work in the 70-84% of HRmax.

Immediate transition from one workout to the other.

When you are done with the total 7 workouts, 1 set is completed.

Rest for 7 minutes and check if your HRmax <50%.
If so, start again another set of workouts.

For achieving HIIT Workout 3, you need to complete 4 sets in total.

HIIT WORKOUTS 3

Number of workouts: 7
Workout Duration: 25''
Set Duration: 175''
Number of sets: 4

Heart Rate Zone: 70-84% of HR max
Workouts Interval: None
Sets Interval: 7' and HR max is <50%
Purpose: Each workout duration is 25'' x 7 workouts (without interval) =175''

HOW TO WORK WITH HIIT WORKOUTS 3

There are 7 workouts

Squat Jump/Push-ups/Triceps in Bench/Lunges/Stair climbing or step jumps/ Burpees/Skipping run (fast) are the seven workouts that you will need for HIIT Workouts 3.

Workout Duration: 25''

You should repeat as many times as you can each workout over a period of 25 seconds for each workout.

Set Duration: 175''

"Duration of each Set is 175 seconds (25'' each workout x 7 workouts = 175'' total Set Duration.

Number of Sets: 4

You should perform 4 sets for a successful HIIT Workouts 3. 175'' seconds of workouts = 1 Set 4 Sets = HIIT Workouts 3

Heart Rate Zone

For best working results, your Heart Rate Zone should be within the 70-84% of the Maximum Heart Rate (HR max).

Interval between Workouts

There are no intervals between workouts. You should rotate from one workout to the other without interval for a period of 3 minutes (3').

Interval between Sets:7'

After you complete a Set (Set Duration = 175'') you can take a break. During the Interval, you regulary check your Heart Rate. When 7' have passed and your Heart Rate is <50% of the HR max, you can continue with the next Set of HIIT Workouts.

Tips:
- use a timer to count the Set Duration (175''),
- rotate workouts every 25 seconds. Do as many workouts as you can,
- the Heart Rate table will help you define your HRmax according to your age,
- if your Heart Rate Zone is higher than 70-84% of HRmax, reduce repetitions until you manage to get your Heart Rate to that Zone. Go back to the original repetitions when you feel ready again,
- interval between sets is really important. Do not start before your Heart Rate is <50% of HRmax.

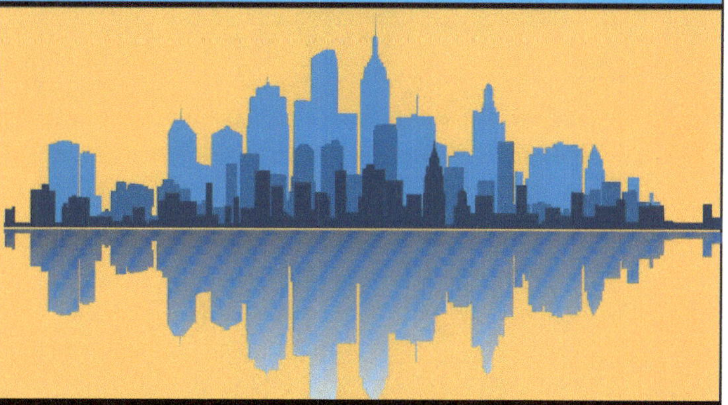

LEVEL 12

MON	**HIIT WORKOUTS 1**
TUE	**LEVEL 6**
WED	**HIIT WORKOUTS 1**
THU	**LEVEL 6**
FRI	**HIIT WORKOUTS 1**
SAT	**LEVEL 6**
SUN	**DAY OFF**

LEVEL 13

MON	HIIT WORKOUTS 2
TUE	LEVEL 6
WED	HIIT WORKOUTS 2
THU	LEVEL 6
FRI	HIIT WORKOUTS 2
SAT	LEVEL 6
SUN	DAY OFF

MON, WED, FRI:
HIIT WORKOUTS 2

TUE, THU, SAT:
LEVEL 6 WORKOUTS

LEVEL 14

MON	**HIIT WORKOUTS 3**
TUE	**LEVEL 6**
WED	**HIIT WORKOUTS 3**
THU	**LEVEL 6**
FRI	**HIIT WORKOUTS 3**
SAT	**LEVEL 6**
SUN	**DAY OFF**

LEVEL 15

MON	HIIT WORKOUTS 1
TUE	LEVEL 6
WED	HIIT WORKOUTS 2
THU	LEVEL 6
FRI	HIIT WORKOUTS 3
SAT	LEVEL 6
SUN	DAY OFF

You can use all HIIT Workouts (1,2,3) in the last LEVEL 15

Notes

Example Notes for Levels 1-6

Days	Level	Push-ups	Triceps	Crunches	Back extensions	Stretching	Activities	Steps per day
MON	6	100	100	100	100	✓	50 min walking	8100
TUE	6	100	80	80	80	✓	30 min cycling	7500
WED	6	80	80	100	100	-	-	12300
THU	6	100	100	-	-	✓	15x2 min running	7500
FRI	6	140	140	160	160	✓	-	2500
SAT	6	-	-	-	-	✓	1 1/2 hr walking	18100
SUN	6	100	100	100	100	✓	-	8300
TOTAL	6	620/700	600/700	540/700	540/700	6/7	4 Activities	64300

Example Notes for Levels 7-11

Days	Level	Front Lunges	Back Lunges	Side Lunges	Squats	Stretching	Level 6	Activities	Steps per day
MON	11	60	60	60	60	✓	✗	1 1/2 h walking	8100
TUE	11	60	60	60	60	✓	✓	-	12300
WED	11	60	60	60	60	✓	✗	30' min running	8100
THU	11	60	60	60	60	✓	✓	-	12300
FRI	11	60	60	60	60	✓	✗	2 hrs cycling	8100
SAT	11	60	60	60	60	✓	✓	-	12300
SUN	11	60	60	60	60	✓	✗	30' min running	8100
TOTAL	11	420/420	420/420	420/420	420/420	✓	3/3	4 Activities	69300

Example Notes for Levels 12-15

Days	Level	Squat Jumps	Push ups	Lunges	Triceps	Stairs climbing	Burpees	Skipping run (fast)	Stretching	Level 6	Activities	Steps per day
MON	12	40	40	40	40	40	40	40	✓	✗	30' min running	10000
TUE	12	40	40	40	40	40	40	40	✓	✓	2 hrs cycling	10000
WED	12	40	40	40	40	40	40	40	✓	✗	-	10000
THU	12	40	40	40	40	40	40	40	✓	✓	-	10000
FRI	12	40	40	40	40	40	40	40	✓	✗	-	10000
SAT	12	40	40	40	40	40	40	40	✓	✓	-	10000
SUN	12	40	40	40	40	40	40	40	✓	✗	-	10000
TOTAL	12	280	280	280	280	280	280	280	7/7	3/3	2 Activities	70000

NOTES FOR LEVELS 1-6

Days	Level	Push-ups	Triceps	Crunches	Back extensions	Stretching	Activities	Steps per day
MON								
TUE								
WED								
THU								
FRI								
SAT								
SUN								
TOTAL								
MON								
TUE								
WED								
THU								
FRI								
SAT								
SUN								
TOTAL								
MON								
TUE								
WED								
THU								
FRI								
SAT								
SUN								
TOTAL								
MON								
TUE								
WED								
THU								
FRI								
SAT								
SUN								
TOTAL								
TOTAL SUM								

NOTES FOR LEVELS 7-11

Days	Level	Front Lunges	Back Lunges	Side Lunges	Squats	Stretching	Level 6	Activities	Steps per day
MON									
TUE									
WED									
THU									
FRI									
SAT									
SUN									
TOTAL									
MON									
TUE									
WED									
THU									
FRI									
SAT									
SUN									
TOTAL									
MON									
TUE									
WED									
THU									
FRI									
SAT									
SUN									
TOTAL									
MON									
TUE									
WED									
THU									
FRI									
SAT									
SUN									
TOTAL									
TOTAL SUM									

NOTES FOR LEVELS 12-15

Days	Level	Squat Jumps	Push Ups	Lunges	Triceps	Stairs climbing	Burpees	Skipping Run (fast)	Stretching	Activities	Steps per day
MON											
TUE											
WED											
THU											
FRI											
SAT											
SUN											
TOTAL											
MON											
TUE											
WED											
THU											
FRI											
SAT											
SUN											
TOTAL											
MON											
TUE											
WED											
THU											
FRI											
SAT											
SUN											
TOTAL											
MON											
TUE											
WED											
THU											
FRI											
SAT											
SUN											
TOTAL											
TOTAL SUM